MW01256847

# Best Sex Ever

## *For Midlife Men*
## *And Their Partners*

## with Daily Cialis

## Erika Thost MD

Published by Erika Thost MD

Copyright © Erika Thost MD 2019
All rights reserved

# Acknowledgements

To my husband Reaps,
And my sons Clancy, Toby and Tristan:

Thank you so much for supporting me in my work.

# Praise for Daily Cialis

"You're in for a treat with Dr Erika Thost's new book! She has a truly deep and delightful perspective on life, well-being, sex, - and men. I don't know how she does it, but she really understands what it's like to be male. Bravo to that! The book has a ton of valuable information that jumps off the page with fun, clarity, wows, and insights you've probably never heard before. Dr Erika Thost's Daily Cialis book belongs on your bedside table as a must-read."
-James Herriot, Ph.D.

"Good to see a woman of passion looking to enhance the lives of men as we age. Pleasure has been disdained by most religious traditions even while they admit God created pleasure. So acknowledging pleasure and passion that does not have to end with the tick of the clock is returning to the oldest truth: God said it was Good."
-Art Andrews, Priest

"Daily Cialis by Erika Thost MD is a wonderfully accessible look at improving sexual happiness, as well as treating erectile dysfunction, effects of aging, loss of libido, and depressive moods in men. With an optimistic and encouraging approach she explores tender topics and proposes an option for increasing libido, sexual function, pleasure and overall joy in life. Dr. Thost is a baby-boomer era proponent of living life fully - a must read!"
-Natalie Horner RN

"I loved Dr. Erika's book Daily Cialis. She really nails what midlife women want from their husbands and boyfriends. She explains with clear and practical instructions how their men can give them great sex - which the men will also enjoy."
-Linda RN

"I think what Dr. Erika Thost is doing for midlife and older men is amazing! Her work for prostate problems is great. Her new book on Daily Cialis for men will help so many men, women, and couples! "
-Barbara Keesling, Ph.D.
Author of *Men in Bed and Sexual Healing*

"Being a guy is harder that it looks! Erika Thost's new book is a real find. Her book is what I needed to be on top of my game every day with more energy, more sparkle and fun. And way better sex!

Reading her book is like she's talking directly to me. Almost like guy to guy, except even better because she's a women who really gets guys. Lots of new ideas and advice that I'd never dreamed of before. I keep her book on my breakfast room table because I'm always looking things up in it. A big YES to Erika Thost's Daily Cialis book! "
-Jaime G., Ph.D.
Scientist
(who likes being a guy even more now)

"I love it! So compassionate, understanding, gentle and inviting. Dr Erika's writing style is so natural and accessible to anyone without talking down or dumbing down. She normalizes and makes comfortable even the most tender topics. I learned a lot! I want every man I know to read this book."
- Z.H., Workshop Leader

"Dr Erika's Daily Cialis book is a rare find: A straightforward, practical guide for addressing medical remediation for sexual challenges, satisfaction and relationship enhancement. I'm grateful to find a candid resource, with cutting edge scientific information, to recommend to the men and couples in my therapeutic practice! The issue is neither rare nor trivial, and this simple, but safe solution is a gift."
-Linda Powers Leviton, MA, LMFT
West Coast Director, Gifted Development Center

"When I turned 70, I noticed that my libido was beginning to fade away. At that time I went to see Dr Erika who started me on Daily Cialis. Within a relatively short time I begin to get my libido back. I am now 73 years old. I'm having more sex with my wife and feeling so grateful to be able to do this at my age. It feels like a gift, and I am ever so grateful. I'm still doing it: Loving life, loving the energy, and loving the connection with my darling wife."
-George L. Yoga instructor and real estate investor

"A powerful book that will truly change your life! About this crucial topic for men: Everything you need to know is in this book!"
-Thomas Reaper MD

"Since I am a somatic sex educator, Daily Cialis caught my attention. At first I was skeptical, but then astonished and grateful when Dr. Thost's information about Daily Cialis helped me to reclaim my senior citizen sex life."
-Joseph Kramer, Ph.D.

"Daily Cialis allows a more spontaneous and natural expression of desire and passion."
-S.B., MD

"This book is a wonderful resource! It combines up-to-date medical information, the expertise of an experienced doctor in her field, and a sex positive and fun perspective on Men's Sexual Health in midlife and beyond. Dr Erika is a great practitioner and brings a unique voice to men and their partners."
-Michaela Boehm, International Intimacy Teacher and Author of *Wild Woman's Way*

"Dr. Erika's book combines honesty and systemic thinking with the medical practice of sexuality - A rare treat. "
-Russell Haber Ph.D

"In my practice I constantly see how erectile dysfunction is such a devastating problem for so many men and their partners. Here, finally, is a solution that is scientific, safe, and easy to do! I'm thrilled we now have a pathway to their finding sexual satisfaction."
-Patti Britton, PhD, Clinical Sexologist, Co-Founder of SexCoachU.com

# Important Medical Disclaimers

*Please read all of them carefully*

- If you think that you have any kind of health problem, please get medical care immediately.

- Never disregard professional medical advice nor delay seeking medical treatment nor stop medical treatment because of something you read in this book.

- Although I am a doctor, I am not your doctor. Reading this book does not create a patient / physician relationship between us.

- This book should not be used as a substitute for the advice of an experienced medical doctor.

## The purpose of this book:

- To inform men and couples.

- To inspire and inform any conversations with your doctor.

- To share my point of view: What I have learned with patients and in the research.

## About this author and Eli Lilly & Co:

- This book is based on the views and opinions of the author.

- This book contains the author's own research and clinical experience.

- This book has not been authorized by Eli Lilly & Co.

- There has been no communication whatsoever between the author and Eli Lilly & Co.

- There have been no financial connections whatsoever between the author and Eli Lilly & Co.

- I use and respect the use of the word Cialis as the brand name that belongs to Eli Lilly & Co.

- The word Cialis is not intended to mean the generic version of tadalafil.

- When talking of the generic version of the drug, the word tadalafil is used.


## This book:

- Is my opinion, based on my experience and research.

- Does not constitute medical diagnosing nor medical advice.

- Does not constitute advice for medical treatment.

- Does not replace the services of your trained health care provider.

- Does not promote nor condone self-medication.

- Does not promise any specific results.

- Is HIPAA compliant in completely protecting patient privacy.

- Contains only case studies that are composites of typical situations but never any specific patient.

## About the contents of this book:

- Always seek your doctor's care first. Go to them with any medical questions.

- The book is intended to promote broad consumer understanding and knowledge about these health topics.

- No warranties nor guarantees nor representations are given about the medical information in this book.

- No warranties nor guarantees are given about the completeness nor accuracy nor timeliness of the information.

- After the book is published new information will come out. Some of it may contradict current research.

- The author is not liable for any damages, loss, or negative health consequences arising from the use of the book.

- References to other sources of information do not constitute an endorsement of them. Use them with the same cautions that are delineated here.

- The book should not be treated as medical diagnosing nor medical advice.

- The book does not include everything that is known about any topic. It only contains a small fraction of what is known.

- Any and all of your medications and treatments need to prescribed and supervised by your doctor.

## For the reader, what you need from your doctor:

- Frequent contact with your doctor or health care provider.

- Ask your doctor about the suitability of any of this information for you.

- Continued up-to-date information from them about your health and about any potential prescriptions for you.

- Continued up-to-date research since the information often changes and gets updated.

- Every man should have a urologist and an internist, and have his health checked by them on a regular basis.

## Your doctor's responsibility:

- Your doctor is responsible for being informed about the latest research and how it applies to your specific health situation.

- The patient and their doctor need to do their own research for any medical situation.

## To the doctors and health care providers:

- This book conveys the views and opinions of the author.

- This book is based on the author's own research and clinical experience.

- This book is not and is not intended to be scientific information for anyone's practice of medicine.

- For the use of Viagra and Cialis and Daily Cialis, the doctor needs to consult the appropriate clinical research, and adhere to the standards of care for the practice of medicine.

- This book is intended solely to inform and inspire conversations with patients, with the public, and with other doctors.

- This book is intended to spread the word and raise awareness about the concept of Daily Cialis.

- However the clinical applications of this concept are still the responsibility of the doctor in all regards.

## More information about this topic:

- is in the chapter on Risks.

- is available in the research on the internet.

- is available from your doctors.

# Abreviations

**DC** - Daily Cialis

**C** - Cialis

**V** - Viagra

**ED** - Erectile Dysfunction

**RE** - Rapid Ejaculation

**DE** - Delayed Ejaculation

**T** - Testosterone

**BPH** - Benign Prostatic Hyperplasia; enlarged prostate

**LUTS** - Lower Urinary Tract Symptoms; bladder and prostate

**HRT** - Hormone Replacement Therapy

**GERD** - Gastroesophageal Reflux Disease

**AASECT** - American Association of Sexuality Educators, Counselors, and Therapists

**SPA** - Sexual Performance Anxiety

**PAH** - Pulmonary Arterial Hypertension

**FSAD** - Female Sexual Arousal Disorder

# Table of Contents

## Nonsexual Benefits of Cialis

## Women and Cialis

## Relationships and Affairs: Cialis and Couples

## How to Do It: Taking Action

# Introduction

## Dr. Erika's Bio

How is Dr. Erika a leading expert for optimal male midlife sexuality?

What makes Dr. Erika your resource for Best Sex Ever?

Why is Dr. Erika the logical choice for a book about this topic?

## Erika Thost MD

- Medical degree from Dartmouth Medical School
- Training in male and female hormone therapy with Dr. Thierry Hertoghe
- Decades of experience as a medical doctor
- Lifelong study of psychology
- Many years' experience in diagnosing and treating middle-aged men
- Extensive research about male midlife health problems
- Specialty training in men's sexuality and sexual problems
- Extensive experience treating sexual issues of men in middle age
- Many years of teaching about male sexuality
- Many years of coaching about male sexual problems
- Her mission: "Midlife men are neglected, and I help them thrive."

## Dr. Erika's areas of study and training:

- Andropause – male menopause
- Sexual issues such as ED (erectile dysfunction)
- The concept of Daily Cialis
- Low libido – low sexual desire
- Lack of drive
- Depressed moods and anxiety
- Low energy
- Decreased competitive spirit
- Effective weight management
- Anti-aging
- Prostate and bladder problems
- Male bio-identical hormone replacement, such as testosterone and thyroid

## Her unique combination of research and experience:

- Solving sexual problems in middle-aged men
- Optimizing male sexuality in midlife
- Testosterone, and other male hormones
- The correct use of Cialis and Viagra
- The correct use of the concept of Daily Cialis
- Methods include sexological and psychological approach
- The combination of body, heart, mind, and spirit in the practice of tantra
- Use of cutting-edge medical and scientific research

## Dr. Erika's mission—and passion—is taking middle-aged men back to being On Top of Their Game!

- Her private practice is in Santa Barbara, CA, and in Oakland, C.
- Her out-of-town patients can be seen via videoconferencing.

## Dr. Erika has created Online Courses:

- Best Sex Ever! Men's Midlife Health and Sexuality
- The Best Sex Ever! nonDiet
- The Best Sex Ever! Happiness Infrastructure Project
- The Best Sex Ever! Singles and Relationship Course
- The Best Sex Ever: Male Sexual Superstars
- Website: DrErikaMD.com

# Why you need this book

What will this book do for you?

Why do you need this information?

How do you want to improve your sex life?

## Case Study:

Jerry is a 66-year-old single, well-educated man who is busy with his work and much loved in his community. However, he was sad about the loss of his erotic self. He is in good physical shape, though a few pounds over his ideal weight.

He has had no sex for four years, and not much in the way of erections for longer than that.

He asks me: "Does getting older have to be this bad?"

On Daily Cialis: He is delighted to feel sexual again! Now he does not feel old but feels like his normal self.

"My relationship to myself and sex has transformed. I am surprised at my erections and sensations."

Since life feels so much better to him, he also feels a renewed will to eat less to drop those extra pounds.

You have a lot of demands on your time.

How do you choose *right now*?

What will give you the most bang for your buck *right now*?

## Check yourself:

- If you have erection problems.
- If you lack confidence about sex.
- If you don't make your lover happy.
- If you are middle-aged.
- If you *feel* middle-aged.
- If you don't know what to do.
- If you let yourself drift downhill.
- If you don't know where to start.
- If you are worried whether Cialis is safe for you.
- If you don't know that Daily Cialis is.
- If you are not having the Best Sex Ever!

Then this book is for you!

## Do you know?

- The ways that Cialis is good for you?
- Whether you are taking Viagra correctly?
- How to take Cialis so it doesn't spoil the moment?
- What to do if Viagra and/or Cialis do not work?
- How to take them for the very best results?
- What Daily Cialis is all about?
- Which myths have misled you?
- What to say to your doctor about this prescription?

## Use the book *your* way:

- Just go for what interests you.

- Pick out the chapters that you need right now.
- Problem-solve precisely for you.
- Because each chapter is a stand-alone information resource.
- This book gets you taking action.
- These actions will give you results.
- They will do it fast.

## The last taboo:

- Do you need to go the bathroom frequently?
- Do you need to go urgently?
- Do you have hesitation?
- Do you get up at night to pee?
- Do you have a poor stream?

Then you need this book!

## You need this information:

- To feel younger and more virile—
- As one of my patients said: "Roll the clock back 20 years!"
- To reverse that middle-aged slide into flatness and blandness.
- To get your life back: From black and white into living color.
- To invest in your future sexual function.
- To learn about prevention of affairs.
- Make the future *you* proud of the present *you* by taking action.

# If You Read This Book...

What will happen if you *do* read this book?

What does this book give both women and men?

What will *you* get from this book?

## Are you a man in mid-life?

Then read this book—or just browse it—to:

- Have the Best Sex Ever now—really!
- Make your lover very happy.
- Re-gain your confidence and cock-fidence.
- Know how to improve erectile dysfunction or ED.
- Improve your urination problems.
- Get all this safely and effectively.

## Are you the wife or girlfriend of a midlife man?

Then read this book—or just browse it—to:

- Enjoy better sex than you have ever had in your life—really!
- Learn about prevention of infidelity.
- Have a lover who has desire for you.
- Have a lover who can perform for you.
- Learn that it is safe for him.

## After reading this book, you will understand:

- How Cialis and Viagra work.

- How they are very safe for almost everyone.
- How to use them for best effects.
- Answers to questions about sexuality concerning Cialis and Viagra.
- How to solve problems with Viagra and Cialis.
- How to make things work better with your partner / wife / girlfriend.
- How to have the best sex of your life now—really!
- Like you never expected when you were young.
- How Daily Cialis improves your overall health.

## For girlfriends and wives: think about:

- What kind of sex do you want?
- Now that the kids are gone, and you have freedom to make love and play.
- Here is the information you need to help you create the sex that you want.
- How you can do that safely, affordably, effectively.
- You can enjoy yourselves with freedom from ED issues.
- You can have intercourse anytime you want.
- How to enjoy quickies or long lovemaking sessions.

## It does sound like Daily Cialis is too good to be true, right?

- How can one pill do all those things?
- This is why I felt compelled to write this book: It really is amazing how Daily Cialis has so many benefits for so

many men. You need to have this knowledge. It is in this book.

- Please feel free to just browse this book: You do not have to read it cover to cover.
- Each chapter is a stand-alone topic. Just browse the chapters that grab you.

# Why I Wrote This Book

## My two compelling reasons:

1) The heartbreak of seeing midlife men silently fading into lifelessness.

2) The delight of seeing midlife men getting back on top of their game!

## It constantly breaks my heart...

...to see middle-aged men—like you—drift downhill into the loss of their real lives. They are not actually dead yet. However, many parts of them are dead and dying. They have given up on their dreams, their vitality, and their masculinity.

It hurts to see this huge waste of potential for the men themselves, for their relationships, for their work in the world. It is a tragedy that the lives of these middle-aged men could easily be so wonderful—but they are not. I cannot bear to see the waste of this precious natural resource.

It is especially painful to watch this because the suffering is so unnecessary! There are tools to "fight, fight, against the dying of the light." The solutions are safe and effective and easy to do.

## Just think what the world would be like...

...if more midlife men felt truly happy, full of energy, and glowing in their sexuality.

...if more men had the energy and confidence to use their life's wisdom for the good of all.

... if more men felt vital enough to pour themselves fully into their lives and relationships.

## You can tell that this is my passion!

Trust me: One does not graduate from medical school and say, "Male midlife vitality is my mission in life!"

## Instead this happened:

In my medical practice, through the years, I observed the men's silent suffering. Gradually I realized the magnitude of this problem. I also noticed the failure of our society to take these men's problems seriously. Our medical system does not effectively take care of middle-aged men.

And, in time, I became fascinated by the hunt for solutions:

The concept of Daily Cialis offers a synergistic way to fix so many male midlife problems, sexual and nonsexual. It is amazing to me how safe and effective Daily Cialis is. However, it does not appear to be widely known and practiced yet.

Can you see why I felt compelled to write this book?

It's time to share my knowledge and experience plus the research.

Can you also see why I feel so much gratitude and satisfaction when my male patients tell me: "Thank you for giving me my life back!"?

## It is time!

- It is time for men to know what is possible, and how to ask for it.
- It is time for doctors to become more familiar and comfortable with the concept of DC.
- It is time for men to stop suffering!
- It is time for the men—and their partners—to have their Best Sex Ever!

# The Concept of Daily Cialis

## Your Sex Life: Naturally Hot Again on Daily Cialis

So, you have gotten yourself into a routine of taking your Cialis on a schedule every day. You have found a good dosage for yourself for now.

- At this point men and couples in my practice often tell me that they are having their Best Sex Ever.
- They are having sex that is more wonderful to them than ever before in their lives.
- They get to use everything they know about sex, and everything they know about each other.
- They can combine all that knowledge with his good sexual function to create something special for themselves.

### Imagine this sexual scenario for you:

- You and your partner can have sex again anytime.
- You can have spontaneous sex and spontaneous quickies because your sexual function is always at the ready.
- You do not have to take a pill and wait before you can have intercourse.
- You feel younger because you function like a younger man sexually.

## Imagine your happier relationship:

- Your relationship is bubbly in a way that it has not felt in years.
- You feel connected and appreciative of each other.
- You are having fun together and enjoying each other.
- You are enjoying the pleasure and the happiness of your bodies.
- Your relationship is enriched by the extemporaneous lovemaking.
- You may feel reminded of your good connections when you were younger.

## Imagine how happy your wife or girlfriend is:

- She also likes the possibility of spontaneity in your erotic connection.
- She feels younger because you are acting younger sexually.
- She appreciates you for making the effort to take the Daily Cialis.

## Imagine this huge benefit of Daily Cialis:

- Sex life feels natural again.
- The sex does not seem contrived or restricted.
- For some women, it just does not feel right for him to have to take a pill before sex.
- For some men, they just don't feel like their vibrant masculine selves when they need to take a pill before intercourse.
- To some people this natural feeling matters hugely.

- To others, it is does not matter at all.
- What is important: For you and your partner to acknowledge and respect your own and each other's feelings on this matter.
- It's also totally okay for the two partners to feel differently on this issue.
- Do make the effort to talk about these topics with each other.
- Let yourselves be surprised to be having your Best Sex Ever.
- And the Best Sex Ever is happening at a time in your lives when you had thought your sex lives would be declining.

## Imagine these feelings:

Now could be your first time to feel the freedom to really enjoy your sexuality:

- Now that the kids are grown and out of the house.
- Now that you feel, "It's now or never."
- Now that you know that you are not getting any younger, and you had better use it or lose it.

## Imagine your better health due to more sex:

- Your health is better because sex is good for your health.
- This holds true for your partner too.
- Regular sex play gives you both:
  - Better immunity, fewer colds.
  - Less stress, less depression.
  - Better sleep.
  - Less pain.

o   Youthful glow.

o   Maybe lower blood pressure.

## Imagine these problems solved:

- DC helps men with the sexual dysfunction caused by antidepressant medication.
- Both of you are sleeping better because you have fewer trips to the bathroom at night due to fewer urinary symptoms.

## Imagine the beneficial sexual effects of Daily Cialis:

- Ability to have erections anytime
- Stronger and more consistent erections
- Increased libido
- Decreased urination problems caused by an enlarged prostate
- Increased testosterone, by a small amount
- Decreased estrogen, which is not good for men
- Improved ejaculatory and orgasmic function

# What Is Cialis?

## The history of Viagra and Cialis:

Viagra was originally developed as a medication for high blood pressure and angina (chest pain due to serious heart problems). When male participants in early research studies reported that they had the happy side effect of increased erections, the research for both Viagra and Cialis shifted to the erectile function.

Cialis was approved in the USA in 2003 for erectile dysfunction. Viagra has been available since 1998. All these medications are by prescription only in the USA.

There have been announcements that Cialis will go off patent in late 2018 and will become available as generic pills. This will bring down the high cost of the pills. Generic tablets are already available in other parts of the world.

## How do Viagra and Cialis work?

Basically, both Cialis (C) and Viagra (V) work by relaxing smooth muscles in the blood vessels and increasing blood flow. In men that includes the blood flow into the penis.

Viagra and Levitra are effective for a couple of hours. Cialis is effective for a couple of days.

Many men worry about getting habituated to Cialis and continually needing more in the future. That does not happen! Cialis will continue to work for you in the same way. Sometimes men do take more Cialis as time passes but that is because they can tolerate more and want the better effects. Or it can also be that, as they get older, their underlying function decreases, and they need more Cialis. But you will never "use up" your lifetime's allowance of Cialis. You can go ahead and use it now—no need to save it for the future.

Men also have concerns about getting "addicted" to Cialis. They worry about having rebound if they take Cialis and then stop. That also does not happen! If you have been taking Daily Cialis, and you stop, you will be fine. You will not have any problems or symptoms. Your erectile function will go back to what it was without the Cialis and no worse. So, it is totally fine to explore the use of Cialis and Daily Cialis. You can start and stop anytime.

## Safety and side effects:

Cialis has an amazing safety record after the gazillions of prescriptions written all over the world for all these years. Some very rare risks are being discussed but some of them are actually not proven to be caused by Cialis. Since men in the age group who take Cialis also tend to be in an age group that has other health problems, sometimes the risk information is confusing. There is more detail about this in the chapter on risks.

Cialis does have some side effects for some men that are not dangerous but can be annoying. Most men have no side effects. The most common side effects are indigestion and heartburn, back pain, and stuffy nose. Just remember that the side effects get better with time, over one to two weeks or more. So, you may want to continue Cialis longer to find out how you feel after your body acclimatizes to the Cialis.

There is more information on this in the chapter on side effects.

## Will I have random erections?

Men also are concerned that they will have uncontrollable erections with Viagra and Cialis. They think that they may end up walking around with an embarrassing constant hard on. That does not happen!

With Cialis and Viagra, you still need sexual stimulation to get hard, just like you need that without C or V. It's just that your body responds more strongly to the sexual stimulation when C is on board. So, you and your partner are still in control when and how the erections happen.

Conversely, if you sit around and watch the sports channel while waiting for the C to make your erection happen, that will not work. If there is no sexy stuff happening, there will not be an erection, even after C was taken.

## Other use for Cialis:

Most people are familiar with C being used for Erectile Dysfunction (ED). However, it is also approved for women and men who have pulmonary hypertension which is high blood pressure in the lungs. For that use, the brand name is Adcirca.

## The overall health benefits as well as the sexual benefits of Cialis:

It reverses many midlife male complaints:
- It improves ED.

- It improves BPH, the symptoms of an enlarged prostate in terms of urination.
- It helps with depressive moods.
- It helps to lower blood pressure.
- It reduces inflammation which causes many health problems.
- It improves blood flow in the heart.
- It improves physical performance at high altitudes. Helps prevent altitude sickness.
- It is used as an anti-cancer medication.
- Relationships are happier.

The information in this chapter is discussed again in more detail in the following chapters.

# The Biochemistry of Cialis

Here we'll talk about the biochemistry of Cialis and Viagra. Feel free to skip this chapter if you wish and jump straight to the practical information about Cialis in the following chapters. Really, the rest of us won't make fun of you.

## The physiology:

Penile erections are mediated by the relaxation of the smooth muscle of the corpus cavernosum and of the arteries and veins in the penis. The corpus cavernosum consists of two sponge-like regions of the penis that fill with blood to create the erection. This process occurs in response to sexual stimulation and is aided by Cialis and Viagra.

## The biochemistry:

Cialis (and, for that matter, Viagra) both inhibit the action of an enzyme called Phosphodiesterase 5 (PDE5), an enzyme that breaks down cGMP; (Ready? That's cyclic guanosine 3'-5'-monophosphate). When the activity of this enzyme is decreased, the level of cGMP in your cells rises.

cGMP is produced as one of the steps when NO (nitric oxide), a fast-acting hormone, is turned on in the body in order to relax the smooth muscle in the walls of blood vessels. Since Cialis slows the breakdown of cGMP, when NO acts to produce cGMP, its levels rise higher than they would without the drug.

And with more cGMP available, the blood vessels widen more. Since this includes the blood vessels in the penis, one is left with enhanced erections. An important note is that Cialis only acts after NO starts the process; sexual stimulation is required to activate the NO / cGMP system in order of for Cialis to do its job. This is why the drug does not cause random, uncontrollable erections.

## A couple of additional notes:

First, don't confuse nitric oxide, the powerful vasodilator enhanced by Cialis, with nitrous oxide, commonly known as laughing gas or "nitrous." These two molecules are distinctly different, and even though their names sound similar, they produce widely different physiological responses.

Second, please be wary of the so-called nitric oxide supplements one finds available online. These are rarely effective; you'd likely just be wasting your money. If you have ED, just to go to your doctor, take the Cialis, and get the most effective treatment.

## The Difference between Cialis and Viagra

When would you choose one over the other?

What is the difference in their effects?

How are the two pills different?

## Viagra

- The generic is called sildenafil.
- It kicks in faster, in about 30 to 60 minutes.
- It is shorter-acting: It lasts for about 2 to 4 hours.
- You can take it up to 4 hours before sex.
- It has to be taken on an empty stomach. If you take it with food in your stomach, it will not do much.
- It is way more effective with little or no alcohol on board.
- It has more side effects in terms of skin flushing, stuffy nose, headache than Cialis.
- Viagra is not used on a daily basis.
- Viagra packs more "oomph" than Cialis: It has a stronger effect for that shorter period of time.

## How do you take Viagra for a dinner date?

- This is the problem that occurs on many dates: You go out. You have a couple of drinks, then you have a nice big dinner with wine. Then you swallow your Viagra and .... nothing happens.
- On dates: I agree with Dan Savage of *Savage LoveCast:* Have sex first! Then go out to dinner after the sex. Sexual function and sexual energy are so much better with an empty stomach and without the alcohol.
- You can take the Viagra before eating. But a big meal will still make it much less effective. So you would eat very lightly. So, yes, men go through a lot of trouble to please the ladies!

## Cialis

- The generic is called tadalafil.
- It kicks in more slowly: It takes 2 to 3 hours to take effect.
- It lasts longer: 1 to 2 days. It is the "weekend drug."
- You can take it with or without food.
- It is also more effective with little or no alcohol on board.
- It has much fewer side effects than Viagra.
- Some side effects, like skin flushing, are less severe than Viagra.
- Some men do notice the side effects of heartburn, flushed face, stuffy nose, and back pain.
- Most people are familiar with taking Cialis as needed for sex. For an occasion where there will be sex or might be sex, then you take some Cialis.
- It can also be taken via a method called Daily Cialis. You take some Cialis every single day, whether sex is planned that day or not. The dosage often is less than one would take for the per-occasion method, however the dosage can be adjusted upwards if needed.
- Daily Cialis has a surprising multitude of general health benefits that are unrelated to the sexual effect. We will talk about that in a later chapter.

## About both Viagra and Cialis:

- They have the same mechanism of action: via the dilation of the blood vessels.
- They both require a prescription in the USA.
- They both cost a lot for the brand name.
- They are about to come out as generics.

- They are already generics in some parts of the world.
- Both may come out as over-the-counter medications in the future.
- They have been on the market for a long time. There have been millions of prescriptions written. So, we have a great deal of information about their amazingly good safety profile.
- The doses that are optimal can vary hugely from man to man.
- Both have the same cautions: Do not use with substances like poppers nor with nitrates for chest pain.

## Occasions when men may choose to use Cialis or Viagra, (even if they usually do not take it):

- For the first time having sex with a new partner
- For sex in a distracting setting
- For sex when he feels there is more at stake or when he wants some help to be able to relax about his sexual function

## Can you get physically addicted?

- You do not get addicted to Cialis or Viagra. If you have used them, you can stop using them anytime without problems. You will not get a rebound effect. Your function will not be worse later because you took these pills.
- You do not get habituated to them. That means that, in the future, you will *not* need more to have the same effect.

- As you get older, and your underlying function decreases, you may choose to use more of them to get the same effect. But that is because your body's function has decreased, not because you are habituated to the drug or that the drug's effect has decreased.

- Both medications could become a psychological habit if they are taken automatically all the time when there is no ED. So don't do that!

## Can I get an embarrassing uncontrolled erection?

- Many men are worried about taking V or C because they fear a constant, uncontrollable erection.

- This is not how these medications work; you still need the usual sexual and physical arousal activities to get hard.

- It's just that the stimulation is more effective with the drugs than without them.

- If you sit around waiting for an erection to appear out of nowhere, then you will be disappointed.

- If you take the meds, and then you get juicy with your partner, you will find your penis responding in a very natural way.

- When the stimulation ends, the erection will subside, as usual.

# What is Daily Cialis?

How would you like to be ready for sex anytime?

Why did you not know that Cialis is safe?

What can Daily Cialis give *you*?

## Case study:

"Dr. Thost gave me information about Daily Cialis last year. I began the regimen shortly after and I cannot think of another single thing in my life that was as effortless and made such an immediate and big difference.

"I did not have any serious sexual problems before I started taking Cialis every day but there has been a terrific increase in my confidence and performance since. I no longer worry about being getting hard enough or staying hard long enough to have tremendously fun, intimate play time with my partner.

"I'm 63 years old and my response has returned to the way it was when I was in my 20's.

"I keep myself fit but there's nothing else I can do physically at the same level I could 40 years ago. With Daily Cialis my partner and I both get the benefit of my years of experience combined with the response and stamina of a 20-year-old."

~Dave

## The development of Daily Cialis:

When Cialis was first approved, it was taken like Viagra and Levitra: The man took it before having sex, on an as-needed basis. And it is still fine to take it that way.

Later on, Cialis was also approved by the FDA for the urination symptoms of BPH as well as ED. The concept of Daily Cialis was created with a dose of 2.5 to 5 mg per day. In this scenario, the man takes the Cialis tablet every day, whether or not there are plans for sex that day.

It continues to surprise me that many medical practitioners are not very familiar with the concept of Daily Cialis. That is why I wrote this book: To get these astounding sexual and nonsexual benefits to more men!

## Why would you take Cialis every day?

You get a steady blood level of Cialis. This does two main things for you:

- You are ready for sex anytime.
- You get the other constant health benefits of Cialis.

## Safety:

Daily Cialis has an astoundingly good safety profile. Serious health events associated with Cialis are extremely rare. And it is unclear whether these events are actually caused by Cialis since the age group that uses Cialis is also the age group most likely to have health problems. There is more information about this in the chapter on risks.

Cialis is also safe because it does not cause habituation or addiction. You can use it intermittently or daily, and you can stop anytime without any problems. There is no rebound or any other adverse effects when you stop taking it.

## Many synergistic benefits:

In my medical practice, I prescribe Daily Cialis for many male midlife men. I continue to be astounded by:

- The large range of problems that are improved.
- The fact that these are sexual as well as nonsexual problems.
- The fact that I just keep finding more and more benefits as time goes on.
- How amazingly effective it is for those problems.
- The fact that, although it is not always completely effective for all men, it definitely works for the vast majority.

There is a synergy of effects from Cialis for many different problems:

- It improves so many problems because the problems— and the solutions—are related.
- For example: Cialis improves erections due to increased blood flow, which also improves general health.

In fact, Daily Cialis has many scientifically proven health benefits, in addition to improved sex:

- It is good for the heart and can help lower blood pressure.

- It functions as an antidepressant.
- It improves the bladder symptoms (LUTS) of prostate problems (BPH).
- When a man takes Daily Cialis, both members of the couple report increased happiness with the relationship.
- The man and his partner sleep better when he has fewer trips to the bathroom.
- It decreases inflammation in the body: That is a huge benefit in many ways because inflammation is the root cause of so many health problems.
- There is more information in the several chapters on the benefits of Daily Cialis.

## The sexual benefits of Cialis:

- Improved erections.
- Increased sexual desire.
- Decreased sexual performance anxiety.
- It can help with delayed ejaculation.
- It can help with rapid ejaculation.
- Somewhat increased testosterone level which is good for men.
- Decreased estrogen level. Estrogen is bad for men.

## Dosages:

Many medical care providers are not yet experienced with the use of higher daily doses of Cialis for better results. Many men do well on 5 mg of Cialis per day. However, many men also need more than that for truly effective function. And, since Cialis is safe, it may be okay to give higher doses to these men. Of course, they do need to be supervised medically to make sure that everything is safe for them.

## Working with your doctor:

Cialis is a prescription medication, so you need to work with your doctor to make sure that you are safe and to get the prescription. If you talk politely to your doctor and have good information, chances are good that they will help you with your request.

There is more information on how to talk to your doctor in that chapter in this book. About working with me: You can get information on my website, DrErikaMD.com.

# How To Take Daily Cialis

What do you need to know to start Daily Cialis?

How do you optimize your Daily Cialis dose?

When do you want your Best Ever Sex to begin?

## Case study:

"It is a Miracle Drug. My erection looks and performs as though I was 18. One thing I did not expect is that it made a dramatic improvement in my pulmonary function both during sex and during hours of sleep. I am happy and alert. I wake up refreshed. Thank you!"

~Randall, 69 years old

## The advantages of Daily Cialis include:

- You are ready for sex anytime.
- Helps with depressive moods.
- Improves relationships.
- Improves prostate health.
- Decreases BPH urinary symptoms.
- Improves your general health.
- Gives you other effects to optimize sexual function.

## How to do it:

Daily Cialis means that you take your Cialis tablet every single day—whether or not sex is planned for that day.

How and when do you take the Cialis pills for the Daily Cialis concept?

- You take a pill every day.
- You can take the pill anytime during the day.
- Take it when you are most likely to remember.
- It is best, but not mandatory, to take it at the same time every day.
- If you forget it, you can take it later in the same day.
- Some men take it in the evening for even fewer trips to the bathroom at night.
- It is best, but not mandatory, to take it with food.
- Some men have some indigestion side effects and prefer to take it earlier in the day, or even in divided doses, with food.
- Some men, especially when they first start, have some side effects of stuffy nose, headaches, and muscle aches.
- These typically settle down as the body gets used to the medication.
- There is more information in the chapter on Side Effects.

## Dosing optimally

Do work closely with your health care provider. Many of them are not familiar with the concept, and with the dosages for DC. So you might want to bring them this Daily Cialis book to make the process easier for everyone.

When you take Daily Cialis, usually your starting daily dose is less than the dose you take for "as needed." The official recommendation is 2.5 to 5 mg per day. However, that is not enough for some men.

Some men need a higher dose for optimal effects. You will get the best effects if you and your doctor try different amounts to find your optimal dosage.

When you find your best amount, that dosage is what works well for your body at this time. However, your optimal dosage may change over time so do keep experimenting. Keeping yourself at the most favorable daily dose will be a most worthwhile ongoing project for you!

## How much Cialis do you take every day?

- The standard accepted dose is 5 mg of Cialis every day.
- This is the exact same formulation of Cialis that you take "on demand."
- It is not a different type of Cialis.
- Some studies actually have used only 2.5 mg of Cialis per day.
- Some men do feel some benefit at the 2.5 mg dosage.
- Some studies have used higher amounts per day.
- The studies have found that the effect is dose dependent.
- That is, you get more effect with higher doses.
- If you are not getting enough improvement, you may need a higher dose.

There is a lot of individual variation in the dosage between men. So don't get hung up on a number but take the dosage that works for *you*!

How can you tell if your dosage is too high or too low?

Look at the chapters on those topics in this book.

## Daily Cialis deserves your serious consideration:

- It may well give you your Best Sex Ever!
- It has done that for many men and many couples.
- It may well turn out to be a powerful anti-aging medication.
- You do not get addicted to Cialis: You can stop at any time with no problems.
- You do not get habituated to Cialis: You will not need more to get the same effect.
- Therefore: You do not need to save your usage of Cialis for later or for "when you really need it."
- You really can have your Best Sex Ever—right now!

# Erectile Dysfunction

How would you like your erections to be improved?

What is your feeling: Is ED inevitable with getting older?

Where are the ways to optimize your own erectile function?

## What is Erectile Dysfunction?

No man has perfect erections every single time. However, if a man's erection issues impact his own and his partner's sexual happiness consistently, then this is ED (previously also referred to as impotence). Fortunately for our generation, we are so lucky to have Viagra and Cialis. They are a huge blessing for so many couples. Can you imagine life without Cialis or Viagra? Just think: The parents of the baby boomers were deprived of the kind sex in middle age and older age that we take for granted today!

In midlife or older men, it is super common for ED to be present to some degree. The statistics are wrong: It is so much more prevalent than the statistics say. For men in their 50's and beyond, most men notice a change in their sexual function to some degree. And, of course, younger men can have those issues too.

In this chapter we will talk about Cialis and Viagra which are the keys for improving ED. We will also talk about other factors to optimize your function. We will also discuss your personal point system to see which factors favor your erections, and which ones impede them.

## What can Cialis do for you?

- The concept of Daily Cialis is usually the best method for solving ED.
- It is convenient and easy to take: You take a pill every day, regardless of whether there are plans for sex.
- DC is reliable, consistent and effective for millions of men.
- But Cialis can also be taken on demand, as needed for each sexual situation.
- It takes 2 to 3 hours to become effective.
- It lasts 1 to 2 days. That is why it is called the weekend drug.
- You can take it with food or without food.
- It has fewer side effects than with Viagra.
- It can also cause a bit of a stuffy nose.
- In rare cases, it can cause back pain: This will resolve as the medication wears off.
- Some men have problems with heartburn when they take it. You can try taking it with food. You can use Prilosec or Tums.
- If you have either of these side effects, it can help to start with lower doses and work up.
- For Daily Cialis the standard dose is considered to be 5 mg. However, many men do better on a larger dose. Talk with your doctor.

## How would you use Viagra?

- You take it on demand, as needed, for each sexual encounter.

- No one cares how many milligrams of Viagra you take. How much men need varies all over the map. There is no point in taking less than the amount that really works for you.

- For men who tend to come before they want to, Viagra can help to lengthen that window.

- You take it on an empty stomach. It is not very effective on a full stomach.

- It is best to allow an hour before it is needed. Although can be effective in half an hour.

- It works better as a preventative than a curative.

- When you are in the middle of things, and the erection is not working: If you take it then, it sometimes works less well than if you had taken it beforehand.

- The effect lasts about 2 to 4 hours.

- "Practice" by taking it by yourself to get familiar.

- Men often get a flushed face—that is normal.

- Men sometimes get a stuffy nose. If it bothers you, just take a Sudafed for that.

- Some men just take a Sudafed along with the Viagra.

- Be sure to get the real Sudafed: It is the one that you get from the pharmacist, behind the counter. The stuff on the shelf does not work.

- Be sure to read up on the risks of Sudafed interfering with urination when there is prostate enlargement.

- Some men actually like to feel the stuffy nose. They like the signal that the Viagra is working. Then they can relax, which supports a positive feedback loop.
- Occasionally men can get a headache. Tylenol or Motrin or Aleve work well for that.
- In rare cases, men will get a blue tint to their vision that resolves when the medication wears off.
- Levitra is another good ED medication that is similar to Viagra. In my practice I have mostly used Viagra, so I am not as familiar with Levitra.

## How do you take Viagra or Cialis for best results?

- When you take them, you are doing that not just for yourself but also for your partner's sake.
- You still need stimulation to get an erection. You will not be having uncontrolled erections. It's just that the stimulation is more effective.
- Again: There is no benefit to taking a smaller amount than your effective dose.
- Often all the strengths cost the same so many men get the stronger pill and cut it. Ask your doctor about that.
- There is no habituation: You will not need more in the future for the same effect.
- There is no addiction: You will be no worse off the times that you do not take it.
- So, there is no need to ration it: Just take it when you need it. Just don't take too much medication too close together.

- The safety profiles of both medications, with millions of people taking them for decades all over the world, are amazingly good.
- They work way better without alcohol. They may not help much if alcohol is on board.
- Be careful about herbal supplements for sexual function. They rarely ever really work.

## Your checklists for prime erectile function:

## Make your best effort for the best results:

- I talk with many men about their sexuality; it is my strong belief that men can improve their erections *more than they realize.*
- However, it does take effort and time to learn about how to have your best erections. So you might as well start now and keep going for the rest of your life.
- You may feel that your erections are sufficient for you to enjoy yourself. However, you may also want to consider whether they are sufficient to pleasure your partner. These are different factors, and both matter.

## Practice good sexual habits:

- Practice your erectile function when masturbating. Take the erections up and down for practice.
- Do not get in the habit of having an ejaculatory orgasm without your best erection.
- Use lube for sex. Always. Plenty. You might as well make it easy to slide in. Plus, the sensations are better for both women and men.

- Pjur or Eros, Original, in the black bottle, is the best lube in my opinion (silicone) because it does not get dry and sticky. Many people use coconut oil or water-based lube but they are not as slippery and do not last as long.

## What helps, what hinders?

- Alcohol use before sex is detrimental, and alcohol over the years is also very damaging. If you want good sexual function, you will need to be drinking very minimally or not at all.
- Do be skeptical of the various pills and potions that are for sale for ED. There are millions of them out there. And they are rarely effective. Likely you'd be wasting your money. Or, if you take something stronger, like yohimbe, the effect is inconsistent and unpredictable. It is more effective and safer to just go to your doctor and get the real thing.
- Drinking coffee regularly is associated with less ED.
- Testosterone works really well for libido. It does not typically improve sexual function right away, but it can help quite a lot over time.
- Don't smoke.

## Are you working your body?

- Do your Kegels. Every day. No more than 100 per day. They make your orgasms stronger too. To do Kegels, you contract your pelvic floor as if you were holding back urine or a bowel movement.
- Exercise regularly and often, with focus and commitment, for better sex for yourself and your partner.

Work out for muscular strength (arms and shoulders, and hips), aerobic capacity, back strength, core strength, and endurance.

- Maintain a good weight. To accomplish that, you need to cut calories. It is an unfortunate myth that you can do lose weight just by exercising.

## What have you done for your prostate lately?

- BPH (enlarged prostate) is not good for erections, so take good care of your prostate.

- Take your Daily Cialis and testosterone for a healthy prostate.

- There is more information about prostate health in the chapter on that topic.

## Your Personal Point System for erectile function:

## How does the Point System work?

- You probably have a sense that some things make it easier for you to get a strong erection. And some things make it more difficult.

- It is definitely worth your effort to identify what those factors or points are for *you*. And to continually keep observing yourself and learning about that.

- In any sexual encounter you want to use your list to maximize your personal plus points and minimize your personal minus points.

- So, do figure out the plus points and the minus points for your own functioning. They will be different for every man. However, there will also be a lot of overlap.

- You may decide to do something super radical: Actually talk to your male friends and learn from them.

## Develop your own Point System:

## These are points that matter for many men:

- The time of day.
- How tired or energized you feel. You can often shift that if you choose.
- Coffee may be helpful.
- No alcohol on board.
- The specific sexual positions: for your turn-on.
- The specific sexual positions: for your physical comfort (back pain is not good).
- The angle of your penis.
- Being at a comfortable temperature: not too hot; not sweating too much; not too cold.
- Which sexy thoughts and fantasies are most effective. Such as: Your thoughts and fantasies about the sex that is about to happen.
- Cannabis (and other substances) may make things more pleasurable for you, however does it enhance or reduce *your* erectile function?
- Use your Kegel muscle occasionally during intercourse.
- Use your mental focus—experiment how that can work for you.
- Do your nipples like to be touched? How?
- Do you have the issue of performance anxiety? More of that in the chapter on that topic.

- Which other factors do you notice?

## Remember that you are complex!

From Marty Klein's website SexEd.org:

"Assuming he's physically healthy, why might a man have trouble getting erect every time he wants to? Here are just some of the reasons:

- He isn't being touched the way he likes (or touched at all).
- He isn't sober when starting sex.
- He's angry at his partner.
- His partner is angry at him.
- He isn't attracted to his partner (for whatever the reason).
- His partner isn't really interested (and may have perfectly good reasons for this).
- He believes he has to have intercourse until his partner climaxes (which his partner may or may not demand).
- He fears the tears or argument that almost always ensues after he doesn't get erect.
- He's in physical pain, or fears triggering physical pain.
- He doesn't expect to enjoy the sex he usually has."

Sometimes you can figure out why things worked better or less well, other times it is a mystery. Men's sexuality is complex!

Do not go gentle into that good night! Fight, fight...for your sexual function to be the best it can be!

# Solve Your Side Effects

How often do side effects occur with Cialis?

Which side effects happen with Cialis?

What will help your side effects?

## Definitions:

Here are the commonly used definitions which we will use here:

- Risk factor: Something that increases that person's chance of a disease.
- Side effect: A secondary, typically undesirable effect.

A side effect with a certain medication is defined as something that is annoying but not dangerous. Most people actually have no side effects with Cialis, or only mild ones. And most of the rest can be managed fairly easily.

Cialis amazingly has essentially no risks! It truly is astounding that Cialis has such an outstanding safety profile! After years of use since 2003 and millions of prescriptions all over the world, there have not been any major risks associated with it.

But it can have some side effects.

## The most common side effects:

- Stuffy nose
- Feeling flushed
- Headache

ERIKA THOST MD

- Back pain, muscle aches
- Heartburn, indigestion, burping

It is important to emphasize that most men are not bothered by any side effects at all. Most men just start the Cialis and are super happy with it, with no problems.

The side effect that men complain about most frequently is heartburn. The next most annoying side effects are the stuffy nose and head ache. Back pain and muscle pain are rarer but still happen.

All these symptoms are due to the medication's presence in the body. They are due to the effect of the blood vessels dilating. If you stop taking the Cialis, the symptoms will resolve as the medication wears off over a couple of days. There is nothing else you need to do. The symptoms will not stay after the Cialis has been eliminated from the body.

The side effects tend to be less for Daily Cialis than for on-demand Cialis due to the smaller daily dose and the acclimatization of the body.

Even if you have severe side effects—if you are willing to be patient and persistent, you can get good results by letting your body get used to the Cialis over time. If your side effects are a big problem, this may take weeks or months. Don't give up! It will be so worth it!

## Dosing for side effects

Most of the side effects are directly connected with the dosage you are taking. Some side effects happen simply because the dose was too high for you at this time. Other side effects are due to how you are taking it, regarding food and time of day.

If you do have these annoying side effects, do *not* power through taking of the medication. Repeat: When a side effect bothers you a lot, it is better to drop back on the dosage for now, than to soldier on and suffer. Later you can gradually increase the dosage as your body gets used to it.

To improve the situation, you cut back to a lower dose. Go as low as you need to feel fine. Then gradually work up to a higher dose by increasing it every one to two weeks. If necessary, you can make the incremental increases very small.

Unlike Viagra, Cialis does not taste bad at all. So, you can cut the pills as small as you need to get your lower dose. Then you can swallow the pieces of the pills. Talk with your doctor about these things.

## If you have side effects, try these things:

- Take the Cialis with food.
- Take your total daily dose of Cialis in two to three divided doses so you are taking a smaller dose each time.
- To do that, take your total daily dose and divide it up by cutting the pill.
- Some men prefer to take it at night because they sleep through most the side effects.
- Some men may get more heartburn if they take it close to bedtime.
- You can even try to take it without food, to see if your body is unusual and does better with that.

ERIKA THOST MD

- You can see that you, as an individual, can figure out what works best for your unique body.

## For more severe symptoms:

- Do keep experimenting with the dosage.
- Some few men do better taking the Cialis only every other day. That way they can tolerate a higher dosage each time. And this works fine since the Cialis lasts a long time in the body.
- Several of the symptoms are alleviated by taking Claritin and ibuprofen with the Cialis: Headaches, stuffy nose, back aches and muscle aches.
- Do follow the instructions for each of those medications.

There are no sacred cows here; whatever you can find, that helps you, is good. Keep experimenting! Talk to your doctor. Talk to other men if you are lucky enough to have close male friends. Your friends may well be using Cialis too.

## For back pain:

If you experience mild back pain on Cialis, cut back on the amount you are taking. Use two to three divided doses and take it with food to slow down the absorption. Use Tylenol, Advil, or Aleve as needed to feel better.

If you experience severe back pain on Cialis, stop taking it for the moment. Do use Tylenol or Aleve or Advil for the pain.

Once the back pain has resolved, usually in a day or two, start the Cialis again with very small doses. Some few unlucky men may need to take just a crumb at the beginning. Take that tiny dose once or twice per day, with food. And still use the pain medications if you need them at times.

## Facial flushing:

Cialis also causes facial flushing various extent in various individuals. Again, the men typically acclimatize over time.

## Stuffy nose:

The stuffy nose is most common with Viagra. Since the tissues everywhere are better perfused, that includes the face and the nose. Viagra also commonly causes the facial flushing for the same reason.

With Viagra, some men sometimes surprisingly find these side effects useful: When they are nervous about their sexual performance, they might welcome these side effects. The flushing and the stuffy nose tell them that the Viagra is on board and is working. So they can relax, which is of course is always a good thing!

Cialis can also cause a stuffy nose. However, it is much less likely and much less severe than with Viagra.

If the stuffy nose bothers you, you can try Claritin or Zyrtec. They are far less likely than Sudafed to cause trouble with peeing. You can also try Neo-Synephrine which is phenylephrine HCl. It is less likely to cause problems because it is applied locally to your nose. You absolutely cannot use this nasal spray on a regular basis because your nose will get addicted to it. Make sure that you check with your doctor about all these medications.

## A potential problem with taking Sudafed:

Some men prefer Sudafed (pseudoephedrine HCl) for nasal congestion. They have no problems with it. However, for other men it causes problems with peeing. Sudafed causes constriction of the blood vessels. Some men who have underlying prostate enlargement may have trouble urinating after taking Sudafed. This problem will resolve as the medication wears off. If you absolutely cannot pass urine, then you need to get immediate medical care.

## If you do use Sudafed:

The Sudafed has to be the kind that you get from the pharmacist behind the counter. This is the kind that requires your signature. The reason for this requirement: It can used for making meth so people need to be prevented from buying large amounts.

The kind of decongestant that is out on the shelves is not as effective.

Only take Sudafed if you have no medical contraindications for it.

Taking Cialis in the evenings can help some men with the congestion. Since they are asleep, it does not bother them.

## Heartburn

Heartburn is also called Gastroesophageal Reflux Disease (GERD) or indigestion or acid reflux.

If you have a history of heartburn even without Cialis, you probably know which foods and drinks are reflux triggers for you. So do avoid those when taking Cialis. You probably also know which things alleviate your heartburn, so you can use those same methods.

The tricky thing about heartburn is that middle-aged men tend to have problems with it already, even without any Cialis. Especially if they are overweight and/or drink alcohol.

So things are complex and confusing. However, it does seem that heartburn sometimes gets worse with Cialis.

To minimize acid reflux: You can take the Cialis in two to three divided doses during the day, and take it with food. You can cut the pill into as many pieces as you want.

You can experiment to see whether Cialis makes your heartburn worse if you take it later in the day, closer to bedtime. For some men, that is true, and they do better if they take it earlier in the day.

Follow the usual recommendations to decrease your symptoms of heartburn:

- Do not lie down soon after eating.
- No eating for the three hours before bedtime! That strategy is also really helpful for weight control.
- No alcohol, at least most nights.
- Stop smoking.
- Don't eat large meals.
- Observe whether these foods are triggers for you as they are for many people: Spicy or fatty foods, caffeine, carbonated drinks.

You can take over-the-counter medicines:

- Proton pump inhibitors: Prilosec or Nexium.

- H2 receptor blockers: Zantac, Pepcid-AC, Tagamet.
- Tums or other antacids.
- Follow the directions.
- Talk with your doctor if you use them frequently.

## Severe side effects

For very rare individuals, the side effects of the Cialis are so severe that they may feel tempted to give up on Daily Cialis. For example, someone could have so much back pain that the Daily Cialis does not feel worth it.

In that case, this is what you do: You take super tiny doses of Cialis.

The dose may be just a tiny crumb cut off the pill. It is okay for the dose to be ridiculously small. Any amount is better than nothing. However, do take the dose every day, except in severe cases, in which case you can take the C every other day. That way the body can begin to both acclimatize to the Cialis and also to get some of the good effects from it. Consult with your doctor about any of the dosage questions.

## Blue vision

Blue vision can happen with both Viagra and Cialis: The world looks as if you have slightly blue-colored glasses on. This effect shares the same pathway as the erectile function: It occurs via the inhibition of PDE6 which is very similar to PDE5 (phosphodiesterase 5). This effect wears off as the drug wears off.

# Risks Of Daily Cialis

The fascinating thing about Cialis is that there are basically no serious proven risks at this time. Considering that this medication has been taken by millions of men and women for many millions of doses, Cialis has an amazingly stellar safety profile.

A risk is something that actually has a negative effect on the human body, where there is the possibility of damage to the body. The only known risk is an arteritis in the eye, which is extremely rare—it occurs in only 4 people per year of the millions of people who take it. That is less than the chance of being struck by lightning.

In fact, as you will see in this book, researchers are constantly discovering new benefits of Cialis and Daily Cialis. There are the sexual benefits of better erections, more libido, sexual confidence, and more. Then there are the prostate benefits of less urgency and frequency of urination, and fewer bathroom trips at night.

Where most of the new benefits are being discovered is the nonsexual arena: It helps with inflammation, depression and anxiety, intra-uterine fetal growth, lung function, high altitude symptoms, and many more. You can read more about them in the chapter on the Nonsexual Benefits of Cialis.

## Here is the short version of the risks—the detailed version is below:

The eye problem called NAION:

With Cialis there appears to be a very small increase of non-arteritic ischemic optic neuropathy. However, you need to keep this risk in perspective: In one year there were four cases among people who took Cialis and got this condition. That is a very small number when you consider that literally millions of people took the medication. That is rarer than the risk of being struck by lightning.

People who have had this condition in one eye, or whose doctors have told them that they are at risk, should not take ED medications. These are extremely rare conditions.

In actual practice, my own eye doctor told me that he has never had to tell a patient not to take Cialis. He has been able to approve all his eye patients to take it. This problem is real and, of course, difficult for the patients who get it. However, his experience shows you just how very rare this problem is.

The recent meta-analysis research papers, when many studies are analyzed to use the aggregate data, report:

- No risk to cardiovascular health. In fact, Cialis is considered to hold promise as a cardioprotective medication.
- No risk was proven for the previously suspected concerns about melanoma, hearing loss, and recurrence of prostate cancer. The data was considered unconvincing and controversial.

## Drug interactions

As is well known, Cialis and Viagra cannot be taken with poppers, which is a recreational drug that lowers blood pressure. They also cannot be taken with the heart medications containing nitrates, which actually are very rare these days. With both of these, the risk is that the blood pressure could drop low enough to cause dizziness, fainting, and possibly death.

As with any new medication, you want to check with your doctor to make sure that they are no risky interactions with your other medications. You also want to discuss the use and dosage of Cialis with your health care provider before you begin and while you are taking it. My recommendation is that you look for someone who is experienced with Cialis and Viagra. Ask your friends: It's time that we start talking about these topics!

## To educate yourself: Use PubMed

You may be more reassured if you do your own research. Believe me, it is fascinating reading! You can do it easily with PubMed.

You put in search terms, such as tadalafil, heart, prostate, depression, etc. Be sure look for *recent* articles. Then focus on the paragraph called "Conclusion" near the end of each abstract.

## Read the following for more detail on risks:

Please note that risks and side effects are different things. In this book they are covered in separate chapters. Risks are effects from a medication that can cause health problems. Side effects are effects that may be annoying but do not cause serious health problems.

Here are the definitions that are commonly used, and that we will use here:

- The definition of risk factor in this book: Something that increases a person's chance of a disease.
- The definition of a side effect in this book: A secondary, typically undesirable effect but not a serious health risk.

When you look at the risks that have been reported with the use of Cialis, you need to be aware of the vagaries of statistics, as well as the overly dramatic reporting style of the media.

Consider the population of men who take Cialis: These are men who are middle-aged or older. They may be taking Cialis because they have diabetes or other chronic conditions which are bad for erections. Men who have heart trouble and many other health issues are going to be men of that age. So it is often difficult or impossible to see whether any adverse effect is due to the Cialis or due to the fact that the men are older and are likely to have these things happen anyway.

Association does not prove causation. This tenet is key to the interpretation of reports of risks. Again, this age group is when health problems happen. And just because the men happened to also be taking Cialis does not mean that the problem was caused by the Cialis.

The news reports often do not give you this information:

When you look at the total number of occurrences, it is vanishingly low compared to the number of men who take Cialis. Of course, if one of those bad things happen to you, then it is a serious problem.

For example: In the past there were reports of sudden loss of vision in men taking Cialis. That sounds really alarming. However, does it sound differently when you hear that the total number reported was 4 men? The number of events was fewer than one in one million. And again, that is in the millions of men and women who take it. And it is in the age group that is most at risk for this problem. So it is worth looking at the numbers.

There are *extremely* rare reports of priapism which is a persistent erection. Typically immediate medical evaluation is recommended if it persists more than 4 hours.

My favorite ophthalmologist or eye doctor tells me that he has never had to tell man that he could not take Cialis due to concerns for his eyes.

Whenever you take a medication, you need to balance the risks and benefits. You have to look at both of them together. It is not useful to look at them in isolation. Cialis has astounding benefits, both for sexual happiness as well as all-around better health. You will read more about that in the rest of this book. So for almost all people, the benefits will be way more than the risks.

This is super important: You, and your doctor, definitely need to evaluate the risks and benefits of taking Cialis for yourself as an individual. You want to go over all your medications to check for interactions. Do your due diligence. Inform yourself from a variety of reputable sources. Wikipedia is usually a good source, as is the official Cialis website, PubMed, and the FDA website.

Then observe yourself carefully. If you have any unusual symptoms, pay attention to them and do not downplay them. Do report them to your doctor. You can look them up on the internet via reputable sources beforehand so that you have some perspective.

If you have any worrisome symptoms, stop the Cialis until you have been evaluated by your doctor. It is always okay to stop taking Cialis. There will not be any rebound or other health problem.

You want to find a doctor who is good at weighing the risks and benefits for you with this prescription. However not all doctors have the experience to optimize the starting dose for you as an individual, and then also to nuance the ongoing dose for you as an individual.

The risks appear to be no higher whether the Cialis is taken as Daily Cialis than when taken as needed. The side effects tend to be less if taken as Daily Cialis due to the smaller daily dose and the acclimatization of the body.

Current research supports the stance that Cialis is either neutral or beneficial for heart health. Some research even seems to show that men on Viagra (similar effect to Cialis) have fewer heart attacks. Research also shows that Cialis may improve the blood supply to the heart which is a good for the heart.

You can always search the Internet for "risks of Cialis" to check on the research that is available at any time. Then, when you choose the websites to read, only choose reputable ones: such as the FDA, PubMed or the official Cialis website.

If you like statistics, you might want to read up in Wikipedia about Numbers Needed to Treat (NNT). You can also do an Internet search on the term for more information. It means: The number of patients that need to be treated for one of them to benefit compared with a control in a clinical trial. The higher the number, the less effective is the treatment. For Cialis it is low. It is 5, which is very good. In fact, one statistical article pronounced a drug with that low of an NNT number as a near-miracle drug. And I agree!

## The following is adapted and quoted from the "Warnings and Precautions" on the official Cialis website:

- I *strongly* recommend that you read the most up-to-date version on the Cialis website.

- Sex is increased work for the heart. If you have serious heart problems, talk to your cardiologist to make sure that it is okay for you to have sex and to take Cialis. Get immediate medical attention for chest pain, dizziness or nausea during sex.

- Do not take it with the nitroglycerin type of medications for angina pectoris heart pain. These are actually rarely used these days.

- Cialis can increase the low blood pressure effects of high blood pressure medications, alpha blockers (including terazosin, doxazosin, tamsulosin, and alfuzosin for BPH symptoms), the recreational drug poppers, and large amounts of alcohol. The symptoms of low blood pressure are extreme dizziness and feeling faint.

- There are other medications that may also interact with Cialis: Alpha blockers (such as for prostate problems), blood pressure medications, HIV or antifungal medications, some antibiotics, other forms of Cialis like Adcirca, and other ED medications.

- There are extremely rare reports of priapism which is a persistent erection. Typically immediate medical evaluation is recommended if it persists more than four hours.
- There have been extremely rare reports of loss of vision or hearing where it is unclear whether they were caused by the Cialis or just happened to occur at the same time. Stop taking Cialis if you experience that.
- Whenever you get medical care, tell them that you are taking Cialis.
- Cialis will not protect you from STD's.
- Cialis does not work as birth control.
- Do not drink too much alcohol, which the website defines as five or more drinks.

## Tell your doctor if you now have or have ever had:

- Heart problems such as chest pain, heart failure, irregular heartbeats, or heart attack.
- Pulmonary hypertension.
- Low blood pressure or high blood pressure that is not controlled.
- Stroke.
- Liver or kidney problems or required dialysis.
- Retinitis pigmentosa, a rare eye disease that runs in families.
- Severe vision loss, including NAION.
- Stomach ulcers or a bleeding problem.
- Deformed penis shape or Peyronie's disease.
- An erection that lasted more than four hours.

- Blood cell problems such as sickle cell anemia, multiple myeloma, or leukemia.

## Now we are back to Dr. Erika:

The above medical problems do not necessarily mean that you cannot take Cialis. In fact, the chances are still good that you will still be able to take it. It just means that your doctor should have this information to have the big picture.

## The bottom line is:

- Educate yourself.
- Talk with your healthcare provider.
- Observe yourself.
- And enjoy yourself!

# Is Your Dose of Cialis Too Low? Too high?

How can you tell whether you are getting enough Daily Cialis?

How safe are the higher doses?

How do you find the best dosage for *you*?

## Case study:

Michael is the classic nice guy who is beloved by everyone and has lots of friends. He is 64 years old. He still works hard as a manager in a factory. He is somewhat overweight and is at risk for diabetes.

His girlfriend had persuaded him to get Daily Cialis from his primary doctor for the ED. He was taking the standard dose every day. His ED was unchanged. He also did not have any side effects which told me that his dose was probably insufficient to have any effect on his body.

We worked together to increase his DC dose safely. It was very clear when the dose was sufficient: Both he and his girlfriend happily noticed that! And, yes, he did have some stuffy nose because the Cialis was actually affecting him now. However he was happy to put up with little nasal congestion in return for his improved sexual function and sexual confidence!

While there is no point in taking more DC than you need, the biggest problem that I see is men *not taking enough* to achieve their desired outcomes. They are worried about taking too much, so they do not go high enough to get the really good results. They

DAILY CIALIS

also do not feel comfortable telling their doctor that they are not
having the full effect.

The dosages for Daily Cialis vary a huge amount between
individuals. And they can vary for you over time.

## The lower dosages:

- Some men do fine on 5 mg per day which is the standard
  dose for DC.
- Some recommendations even call for 2.5 mg per day as a
  starting dose for DC.
- Some men need higher doses.

## When to use low dosages:

- The very low doses can be useful for the rare man who
  has severe side effects such as back pain or indigestion.
- In those cases, one may need to start literally with just a
  crumb of Cialis per day, or even just every other day.
- Then try to gradually increase the dose as the body
  acclimatizes.
- The important part is to take the dose regularly so that
  the body can get used to it over time.

# When to ask your doctor about maybe increasing your dose:

## Regarding erections:

- If you are not getting enough effect for your erections: If they are not firm enough, if they are not reasonably reliable, if they do not last long.
- No man has perfect erections every time. So don't aim for that.
- If ED is still an issue and if you are *not* getting side effects, that may mean that your dose of Cialis is too low to have any effect on your particular physiology.

## When to ask regarding other problems:

- If you have other sexual issues such as delayed ejaculation or rapid ejaculation, and you want to see how much improvement is possible.
- If you have low libido, and you really want to get that back as much as possible.
- If you have issues such as depressive moods, and you want to see how much better you can get with Cialis.
- If you want Cialis for a special purpose: Such as high altitude physical performance.
- If you take a lower dose of Daily Cialis every day, and you want to try taking more before having sex.
- As you get older, you may need more medication since the underlying function is dropping.
- Your doctor may be okay with a higher dosage as a temporary trial.

## Why are men, and their doctors, hesitant about the higher and more effective doses?

- Maybe there is a bit of puritanism going on.
- Maybe there is something like "We can't have these men having too much fun."
- Maybe there is a feeling of "It is not okay to focus on sex that much."
- Maybe men worry that they will "have to pay" for having too much fun.
- Maybe the men and their doctors are not comfortable talking about the details of his sexual function.
- Maybe there is worry about safety.

## Are you worried about safety?

- Cialis has an amazingly excellent safety profile for the millions of prescriptions the world over. There really are no serious risks for almost all men.
- It is important to use your critical thinking, and your knowledge of statistics, to evaluate how this information impacts your individual risk.
- Some of the worrisome incidents occurred in so very few men that it is hard to assess whether there was a possible connection with the Cialis.
- Also the men who take Cialis tend to be of the age where health problems happen more frequently, with or without Cialis.
- When you search the Internet for the risks of Cialis, be sure to consider the source. PubMed is good.
- Only read information from serious and credible sources.

- Be sure to also read the chapters on Side Effects and on Risks.

## On the other hand:

## How to tell if your dosage is too high:

- If you just don't feel right in general, and you feel better at a lower dose.

- If you get a lot of side effects that really bother you, such as a stuffy nose, indigestion, or back pain.

These are not dangers but can definitely be annoying.

## At the doctor's office:

- Gather all your information before your doctor's visit so that you can communicate clearly with her or him.
- Have your questions written out so you don't forget any of them.
- Give precise information about that the problem. Don't be shy.
- Be straightforward about what you are requesting.

# Effective Sexual Stimulation

Which kind of sexual stimulation works best with Cialis?

What can the woman do for more erection action?

How do you do Male Genital Massage?

Both Viagra and Cialis do an amazing job for a vast number of men. Some men just need to pop the pill and are set to go. However, some guys need a little more finesse for the Cialis to work best.

For the best effect, remember that Cialis needs focused sexual stimulation. Although all men enjoy this focused stimulation, some men need it more than others. If you are one of these guys,

- You need the sexual stimulation to be more focused, and
- You need the erections to be used right away.

## Effective sexual stimulation:

Are you getting enough sexual stimulation to encourage the erection? It is still needed to get hard. You cannot just swallow the C or V and then sit down and watch the ball game, waiting for the erection. You will be waiting for a long time because this is not how these pills work.

With both Viagra and Cialis, your body functions like normal in terms of responding to sexual stimulation: Your erection happens because there is erotic touch to your body and your genitals.

The V or C just shifts things so your body responds better to the arousing foreplay. But you or your partner still need to supply the stimulation for your penis and for the rest of you to get aroused.

This foreplay can be both the man receiving the stimulation, as well as the man giving caresses to his partner. Both giving and receiving are a big turn on for him. Many men find it incredibly exciting to give oral sex to their partner and watch her get turned on. He loves watching her orgasm. He can be stroking his penis to get hard, while he gives oral sex. Don't rush that part of the sex play!

So, for optimal erections, make sure that his whole body gets touched and caressed. This should be followed by hands—or hands and mouth—on his genitals. Show your lover how you like to have your penis and scrotum touched. Many men like the touch on the penis to be quite firm, so you may need to show your partner that it really is good to give you firmer touch. It is also totally fine for you to get yourself hard.

## Male Genital Massage

One great way for the man to receive arousing touch is Male Genital Massage. You can find some good instructional videos on YouTube. Male Genital Massage is using both hands on his genitals to provide pleasure and arousal. It is different from a hand job. A hand job uses repetitive motions to produce an ejaculatory orgasm. In our situation here, we want the turn-on, but we do not want the orgasm yet.

The key to Male Genital Massage is using varied motions, not the same one over and over. The hands—with plenty of lube or lotion—move up and down and around the penis. Swirling motions are wonderful. Soft touch and slow touch are wonderful. You can get very creative here!

## Important hints about Male Genital Massage:

- The massage strokes on the penis should be slow to medium fast.
- Vary the speed.
- Don't go fast. Do not speed up.
- When going from the base of the penis towards the tip, you can use touch that is quite firm.
- When going form the tip to the base, you want lighter touch to make sure that you do not bend the penis by mistake.
- Use both hands.
- Use lube or plain lotion. Use something that will be okay inside her vagina later.
- Some men prefer lots of lube for smoother touch. Some men like less lube to feel more friction.
- Use swirly motions, not just up and down motions.
- Focus on the head of the penis, on the corona, and on the frenulum. The corona is the ridge around the lower edge of the head of the penis. The frenulum is the looser skin just below the corona on the underside of the penis.
- Use varied motions, not repetitive.
- Ask the man how he likes his testicles and scrotum touched. There is huge individual variation there. Be sure to be very gentle on the testicles!
- Make sure that the giver of the genital massage is in a very comfortable position ergonomically so that her back does not hurt. Maybe she can lean against the headboard.

Keep experimenting to figure out what kind of foreplay turns you on. Those things can change over time. Some men also respond to sexy talk, sexy videos, or kinky play. Many men find nipple play, with light or hard pinching, to be very arousing.

Some men like to be touched on the outside of the anus. Many men also like a finger or a toy inside the anus and on the prostate. Please look at my book *Sexy Prostate* for easy instructions for that. Basically, all men are curious about anal pleasure and prostate massage. And most men love it. Plus you get an added bonus: The prostate massage hugely helps the man's prostate health and sexual function.

It is important to note that many men need a long time of very intense stimulation to produce an erection. This is true even with the Viagra or Cialis on board. So please don't give up on V or C if you have not really given foreplay some serious focus.

## Women, use the erection right away

When the erection happens, use it right away! Don't waste it!

With some men, there is lots of time: The erection will stay or it will come back. However for many men, the erection may not stay long if it is not used. So the female partner has to be physically and mentally aroused and ready to go so that she can enjoy the intercourse when his penis is ready.

Earlier in life, it may have worked fine to have the women determine the cadence and the pacing of the sexual encounter. It was usually her rhythm that determined the length of the foreplay and the timing of the intercourse. However, now that she has a midlife partner, the situation may be reversed: If you both want sexual intercourse, she needs to learn to be ready when the penis is ready. If she waits, the erection may fade, and then it may or may not return.

## The first erection is the best

One thing that many women may not realize: The first erection is the best. Usually the first time that a man gets hard, his penis is the hardest that it will be for that session. Subsequent erections typically are less hard and less dependable. So be ready to use it right way! Don't waste it!

## How she can get aroused to use that first erection

This situation is not as harsh as it sounds: The woman can easily learn to produce much of her own turn-on. These things are actually validated by research about women who like a lot of sex. You can look it up on the Internet.

One way is to play with sexy thoughts before love making even starts. Another way is for her to get sexy touch by hands or mouth or vibrator early on to get her aroused. This may also start with her own hands on her body, breasts and genitals before the official sex date starts. It can begin with kisses and hugs earlier, even before the sex date.

## Vary the routine:

Yes, we get really good at using a routine for "getting each other off" after we have been together for a few—or for many—years. And there is nothing wrong with that. There also is nothing wrong with quickies which focus on being goal-oriented to get either or both of the partners to orgasm.

However you also want to keep exercising the muscle of non-routine sex. Don't always follow the routine of: Kiss, breast, pussy, her orgasm, penis attention, intercourse, his orgasm. The activities we call foreplay are great at the beginning of sex but do them at other times too, not just in your regular routine sequence of the sexual encounter. Don't just use foreplay for foreplay—let it also just be erotic play for anytime.

## A quickie can be great!

It can be really fun and really intimate and really hot to have a quickie:

- Perhaps it's focused just on one partner receiving nonsexual and sexual pleasure.
- Maybe only hands are used, for genital massages for one or both partners, without having intercourse this time.
- Maybe it's a session of kissing and making out.
- Maybe the man brings the erotic energy up and bubbling, but he does not have an ejaculation.
- You may end the quickie when your energy is still high.
- You can "both take that erotic energy and turn it into energy for life": You use it to cook a fabulous dinner, run a dynamite meeting, write a rocking chapter for your book, have a great work out.

# Cialis Not Working? The Mental Part

When have you felt that Daily Cialis is not working?

Where have you given up on your erections?

Which approach gives you more effective action against ED?

Daily Cialis and as-needed Cialis create better erections for the vast majority of men. However, unfortunately that is not true for all men. In this chapter you will get information about what to do if you are not getting good results.

## Daily Cialis is not giving you better erections?

## Check on these things:

- Keep the DC going for a while. Sometimes it can take a few days or a couple of weeks to really become effective.
- Do you consistently look to learn more about sex and sexual function? Watching porn does not count as learning.
- If side effects are a problem, review that chapter in this book. Side effects are solvable.
- Have you given up on solving your ED?
- Are you living with semi-functional erections but not motivated to improve more?
- Do you have beliefs that keep you from taking DC?
- Do you have fears that keep you from taking higher doses?
- Discuss these issues with your doctor.

- Find a doctor who is experienced, who takes your situation seriously, and who talks with you about your progress.

## Do not resign yourself to your ED situation!

- I see this all the time: Men give up on working to improve their function.
- They do not even realize that they have given up.
- They do not really put in the time and effort to learn more.
- They do not consistently take action.
- Their actions do not show commitment to solving this problem.
- To make progress, you would commit to the items in this chapter plus other ones in this book.
- I see this even with patients in my own medical practice:
  - o Then it's my job to inspire them to see what is possible.
  - o And it's my job to create an action plan to move them in that direction.

## A sneaky but common problem:

Unfounded fears, toxic beliefs, and damaging myths:

- Do these worries keep you from taking your optimal dose of DC?
- Do you have a fear of taking Cialis?
- Do you have fears of taking prescription medications?
- Are you worried about vague future problems due to taking Cialis now?

- Do you feel that it is wrong and dangerous to take pills?
- Are you okay taking supplements but not "real" medications?
- Do you feel that you "should" be able to solve this problem with the perfect diet?
- Or the perfect work out regime?
- Or the perfect meditation practice and enlightened state of mind?
- Or the perfect detox or cleanse?
- Do you feel that you "should" only need a small dose of C?
- Do you feel that taking a larger dose of C means that you are a failure?
- Do you believe that you "should" not focus on sex so much now that you are older?
- Do you notice that you do not permit yourself to spend money, energy, and time for a good sex life?
- These are unfounded fears, toxic beliefs, and damaging myths that deprive *you* of good sexual function.

## Move towards a constructive and rational attitude:

- Use PubMed and other sites to research your concerns and fears.
- Be aware of media hype. Check the validity of their science.
- Carefully choose your sources of information.
- Read the chapters about the risks and side effects of Cialis.
- Be aware of peer pressure in your social circle.

- How does peer pressure affect you in ways that are subtle and difficult to see?
- Choose to question authority. Especially your own.
- Just make up your mind to stop being irrational, emotional, and fearful.
- Just do it: Be logical and scientific.

## Keys to improving your sexual function:

- Constantly learn more and take action.
- Be a researcher about your erections.
- Find your Personal Point System from the ED chapter and note: Which factors give you a better shot at good erections? Which factors are negatives for you?
- Those factors could include: Feeling hot or cold, alcohol, food, sexual positions, your own thoughts and fantasies, stroking yourself in certain ways, and many more.
- Experiment and practice by yourself when masturbating. Which touch and which fantasy work for you?
- When masturbating, try to come only when you are at your best erection.
- Be committed and serious about studying yourself that way.
- Observe yourself and learn.

## You need the right doctor!

- Find a doctor who is really experienced in this problem.
- Find someone who takes your situation seriously.
- Be willing to make the effort to find this doctor.
- Be willing to spend the money.

- Be willing to travel or have the visits take place via videoconferencing on your lap top.
- Do not settle for someone who does not specialize in this field.
- Do not settle for someone who sells you a ton of supplements and a radical diet.
- Do not settle for someone who blames *you* for lack of progress.
- Do not settle for someone who is uncomfortable talking about the details of your sexuality.

## Optimize your erections in these ways:

- Do remember that sex goes better without a lot of food in your stomach.
- Do *not* obsess about the perfect diet. Unless your diet is very bad that will not make that much difference.
- Do not obsess about the perfect supplements and vitamins. They do not make much difference.
- Do not obsess about the perfect workout regimen.
- As long as you get some regular exercise, you are fine in that department.
- It does help to be physically fit so that you can stay in sexual positions without discomfort or tiredness for a long enough time.
- Don't be overweight. To attain a good weight, moderately reduce your caloric intake. Exercise alone does not work.
- Look at Brian Wansink's books and website for painless ways to eat and drink less. It really works.

## What really makes a difference?

- No alcohol. Either no alcohol or one (small!) drink will optimize your function that day or that evening.
- Minimizing your alcohol intake every day will optimize your sexual function and your libido over time.
- Have several days per week with no alcohol.
- Alcohol is poison for midlife men.
- Do your Kegels: Exercise your pelvic floor muscles by contracting and relaxing them. 10 sets of 10 quick contractions plus 10 long contractions to the count of 10 is a good amount. Don't do more than that. Be sure to relax fully at the end and periodically in between.
- Read about ED in this book.
- Consider sex therapy with someone who is experienced and action oriented.
- Typically sex therapy will be way more successful when accompanied by testosterone and DC.
- Find a sex therapist via AASECT.
- Set up realistic expectations; it is unlikely that you will have a constant rock-hard erection in situations that are distracting or stressful.
- Make this your focus: Have fun! Enjoy yourself. Enjoy your partner. Create hot and sweet scenarios for the both of you.
- At the time when you want to get hard, learn to contain and focus your sexual energy: Don't be all over the place.
- Really radical: Talk to other guys. Ask them what works for them. This works best in one-on-one situations.

- If they say that they never have that issue, they're not comfortable with that conversation. So move on and ask someone else.

## Consider adding testosterone:

- DC and testostcrone (T) have amazing synergistic effects: Both together do way more than one would expect.
- Sometimes when you don't get much response from CD, adding T makes a big difference.
- Sometimes when you get don't much result from T, adding CD makes huge difference.
- Make sure that the dose of testosterone is high enough to be effective.
- Of course, you would only use testosterone under the supervision of an experienced doctor.
- You would only use it if it is clinically indicated for you and safe for you.
- Testosterone can improve sexual function over time. It can take a few months to being to see the improvement.
- However if your ED is severe, then it helps to add in all possible factors that can help.

# Cialis Not Working? The Nuts and Bolts

What have you not done yet to optimize Daily Cialis for yourself?

Where are you not taking Cialis correctly?

How can make your Cialis work better?

## Case study:

Thomas is a 66-year-old retired real estate agent. He knows everyone in town and seems like a happy guy. He is very social, so he goes out almost every night —and consequently he eats a lot and drinks a lot of alcohol. He is somewhat overweight.

When he came to me, it was heartbreaking to hear how he had not been able to have an erection for years. He and his wife missed that terribly.

He had been taking some Cialis off and on, in random dosages. However it had basically no effect on him at all. Interestingly he also had no side effects from it.

When I started him on DC, we had to work together for a while to get him up to the dosage of DC that started to be effective. He needs a higher dose. Interestingly, on this dose he does note some nasal stuffiness which indicates that the C is actually active in his body.

He is also willing to have only two drinks maximum per week. I gave him some other pointers for improving their sex life, which he implemented. Now they are able to have sexual

intercourse almost every time they have sex. They never
expected to have a sex life again, so they are very happy!

## Cialis not working? Check on these factors:

- Not taking enough Daily Cialis.
- Not taking it correctly.
- Check for problem medications.
- Get a medical checkup.
- Not enough effective sexual stimulation.
- Low testosterone.
- For some men, C or V really are not going to work:
- They may need vacuum pump, injections, or implants.

## Not taking enough DC?

- You might not be taking a sufficient amount.
- There really are no standard doses of Viagra and Cialis
  because men are so different from each other.
- How can you tell that you are taking enough?
- Interestingly, your side effects can help you determine
  your optimal dose.
- If you are taking a regular dose of Cialis but are not
  getting any ED improvement from it, check to see if you
  are having any of the side effects.
- Because, if you are not having side effects, then probably
  you are not getting the main effect either.
- If you never explore how you do on higher doses, then
  you will never know whether the erection meds just don't
  work for you.

- Or whether you just are one of those men who needs a higher dose for some reason.
- You and your doctor need to talk about the optimal dosing for *you*.

## Are you taking Cialis correctly?

- Make sure that you take it early, with plenty of time before it is needed: 3 hours or more.
- This is a good reason for taking Daily Cialis: You don't need to worry whether you are taking it at the right time.
- Try taking it without any alcohol on board: Zero, nada, none.
- Also try taking it after not drinking any alcohol for a longer time—like a few weeks. Alcohol is an erection killer, both in the short term and in the long term.

## Check for any problem medications:

- Always research the side effects of all medications that you take: So many of them impact sexual function negatively. Be politely assertive with your doctor to try alternatives.
- Medications that can affect sexual function include the alpha blockers—such as Flomax—for prostate problems.
- Some blood pressure medications can be a problem.
- If you have mild borderline high blood pressure, you and your doctor might consider a trial of Daily Cialis. Cialis and Viagra have some effectiveness in lowering blood pressure. Viagra was originally developed as a medication for high blood pressure.

## Get a medical check-up:

Go in to your doc for a visit, even though only rarely is a medical cause found, such as diabetes.

## Effective sexual stimulation:

- If you do not fully provide the foreplay, then you might not get the best response from the Cialis.
- Do focus on high-quality, individualized, arousing foreplay.

## Testosterone and Daily Cialis together provide a powerful synergy!

- If Testosterone (T) is restored to an optimal level, it can help C to work best.
- Testosterone and male sexuality are more complicated than people commonly believe.
- Testosterone actually is safe for most men.
- Testosterone levels drop in all men at some point in their lives.
- In midlife or older men, testosterone levels tend to be lower.
- Low T levels affects men's sexuality and general well-being in many ways.
- More info about testosterone in the chapter on that topic.
- T therapy has its most dramatic effect in repairing low libido: The man gets his sexual desire back, and also his spark in life and his confidence in his masculinity.
- T typically does *not* help much with erection issues.

- This is contrary to what people expect. People mistakenly believe that T improves all sexual function.
- Although, over months of T therapy, sometimes there is some positive effect on ED.
- For the erection issues, DC needs to be added to the T therapy.
- Those two therapies together are dynamite! There is a strong synergy of T with DC.
- T needs a prescription.
- And you need a doctor who really knows this field.

## The power of synergy:

Some men who initially had a poor response to V or C, but then had their T level restored, found that V and C did work after all.

## Do V and C really not work at all for you?

Before you put yourself into that category, check out these factors:

- Try every one of all three different drugs: Viagra, Cialis, Levitra.
- New ED drugs may come out—try them too.
- Talk with your doctor about doing an experiment with higher doses.
- Get your testosterone to an optimal level with prescription testosterone therapy. And keep it there over time.
- Get your estrogen down to a good low level. Estrogen in your body is your enemy.

- Experiment with focused, energetic, and long foreplay.
- Experiment with no alcohol for several months.

## Devices and other modalities for ED:

If you are doing all these things, and the erections are still not working for you and your partner, you might consider adding other modalities:

- Some men like the vacuum pumps to get themselves hard. You can just buy them from places like Amazon.
- Some men find injections useful. These are injected directly into the penis with a tiny needle. It can be a single medication. Or it can be a mix of two or three medications. These prescriptions are usually given by a urologist.
- Another medication can be applied as a tiny urethral suppository. This prescription is also usually given by a urologist.
- Another option is a penile implant. This choice is something that you would discuss with a urologist.

## More power of synergy

- Even if DC does not produce full erections, it can still help optimize these other modalities.
- When you use these other devices and modalities, still be sure to maximize your testosterone and DC dosing.
- These medications may give you some improvement in function over time.
- Plus, they help with libido and other important factors.

- Don't just take any random low dosage of them because you assume that it won't do much good anyway.
- Work with your doctor. Figure out your optimal dosages and be consistent in their use.
- You might as well have *all* the factors going for you, for the Best Sex Ever for yourself and your partner!

# Specific Sexual Issues

## How Can You Have Your Best Sex Ever?

How can men really have the Best Sex Ever when they are over 50?

What makes it the Best Sex Ever?

Why is that possible even for men in their 50s and 60s?

## Case Study:

Jim is a dynamic 53-year-old man who is in great physical shape. He is busy and involved with business, hobbies, and outdoor activities. When he first came to me, he felt that that he was aging and that his masculinity was fading because his sexual desire was so low. He was suffering from depressive moods. Life felt flat. Also, his erections were not sufficient to have sexual intercourse.

After he was started on Daily Cialis, he was very happy with his erections. On the combo of DC and testosterone, he bounced back dramatically on all fronts. His moods became upbeat and positive again. He was happy to feel sexually juicy and awake. He felt that his erections and orgasms were best ever since he was a young man. He told me "You turned the clock back 20 years!"

He is having his Best Sex Ever!

## How can you have your Best Sex Ever?

These are the main reasons that you can have the best sex of your life in your 50's and 60's:

- You have lots of life experience, as we discuss below.
- You have information about and access to Daily Cialis.
- You have information about the benefits of testosterone, as discussed in that chapter.
- You have information about keeping your prostate problem-free, as discussed in that chapter.
- You can have Best Sex Ever even beyond your 60's!

When we are young, we tend to assume that "old people" do not have sex. It seems obvious that when those bodies look older and function less well, then sex would just fade away.

When we are older, sometimes we assume that young people with their nice taut bodies must be having the most dynamite sex all the time. And we definitely don't expect that for us middle aged people. However young people also have sexual issues, and older people also have tons of fun.

Many of us are completely surprised when sex is still great in our fifties, and then in our sixties. We totally did not expect this when we were young. And then we are surprised that not only is it still great, but actually it is the Best Sex Ever.

## Let's figure out:

- What makes it the Best Sex Ever?
- What can *you* do to optimize your chances for your sex life to the best it can be?

- What are the possible pitfalls? They are discussed in the chapter on that topic.

## Middle-aged people's life in general is the "Best Ever" because:

- They are in the fullness of their rich life experience.
- They have gained perspective on what's truly important. And what is not.
- They have learned a lot about themselves, and they use that information.
- They have figured out how to manage themselves to be happier in their own skin.
- They have learned a lot about nurturing relationships.
- They know how to listen to women, and how to talk to women.
- They have realized that they will die.
- And therefore, they are willing to make more effort and take more risks to live life to the fullest.
- They have "arrived": In life, in their work, in their accomplishments.
- They are quietly confident in themselves.
- They have more time because the kids are grown up, and work is less consuming.
- They have more physical space and privacy because the kids have left home.

## Midlife sex is the best ever for many men and women because:

- They translate the life experience from the list above into their relationship life and their sex life.
- They have a lot more sexual experience now than they had as a young person.
- They have done, and are constantly doing, more sexual learning.
- They have the time, energy, money, and curiosity to keep learning about sex and about relationships.
- They have learned and are constantly learning sexual tools and skills.
- They are more uninhibited.
- They are ready to break loose and explore more aspects of sexuality.
- They have the maturity to slow down and enjoy.
- They are less constrained and are more willing to venture into the more adventurous areas of sexuality.
- They realize the finite-ness of life. And so they push themselves to look at their dreams and fantasies with more focus
- And they also do that for their partner's dreams and fantasies.
- They become more free-spirited in many ways.

## To optimize your sex life in midlife:

- Seriously consider Daily Cialis.
- Consider testosterone for yourself.

- Find a medical practice such as my medical practice: Someone who *really* knows this material who will have your back for optimal midlife health and sexuality. Then make appointments often enough to continually optimize.
- Create peak sexual function for yourself. Observe yourself: What improves your sexual function? What diminishes it?

## To optimize your physical well-being for better sex:

- Stay in good physical shape. Find ways to move your body that you don't hate.
- Eat lightly to keep your weight down. However, do not waste too much time and energy obsessing about the perfect diet.
- No alcohol. Or just minimal amounts on just a couple of nights per week. If you cannot do minimal use of alcohol, just stop it completely. It's poison for you.
- Not too much use of cannabis either.

## To optimize your dreams-and-schemes aspect of sex:

- Be willing to spend the hours of time and the emotional energy to identify your fantasies and dreams.
- Take steps toward making them happen.
- Do the same thing for your partner's fantasies and dreams.
- Educate, educate, educate! Continually educate yourself about all aspects of sex: Buy and read books, hire people, take courses, go to workshops.

- Try new stuff and observe the results—in yourself and your partner.
- Focus on fun!

For the nuts and bolts on using Daily Cialis, which is the most effective tool for the Best Sex Ever in midlife, go to that chapter in this book.

# How Is Your Libido?

How do you know if your sexual desire is low?

How do you get your libido back?

Why does better sexual desire make men happy?

## Case Study:

George is a quiet, intellectual man in his 50's. He is a college professor who loves his work and is recognized in his field.

He noticed that his low moods and anxiety made his life less wonderful. He did not have severe depression, but he did have many symptoms of depressive moods. He has also noticed that his erections were less firm.

He had read up on his symptoms and had decided that he wanted to do something about them. He did not want to live the rest of his life feeling like this.

He got started on the proper doses of Daily Cialis and testosterone for him. He was amazed that his moods lifted noticeably. The depressive feelings were completely gone with this treatment. The firmness of his erections returned to the same level as in his younger years. He is very happy that he took action!

## Libido is sexual desire:

- It is the awareness that you are a sexual being.
- It means that you have a juicy appreciation of attractive people in your world.

- You periodically think about sex.
- You fantasize about sex and sexual situations.
- Those fantasies are pleasurable and exciting.
- You like the idea of sex.
- You look forward to having sex.
- You make the effort to create situations for sex.
- You believe that good sex is your birthright and deserves effort.
- You spend energy and money to create sensuality and sexuality in your life.
- And this energy, money and intention also serves you to have better sex.
- Libido applies to women as well as men.
- Although here we are mainly talking about men.

## The positive feedback loop:

- You love making the effort. Your efforts lead to more fun and connection, which gives you that empowered feeling in the world, and that in turn encourages you to keep making the effort.
- There is another positive feedback loop: When a man has sexy thoughts or sees attractive visuals, he responds to both with a juicy feeling. And he may also feel a "stirring in his loins." And those juicy feelings plus body response feed his libido. And when a man has a strong libido, he is more likely to think sexy thoughts and notice the attractive visuals.

## Let's be clear:

- Sexual desire in a woman or a man is a pure and wonderful feeling.
- We can fantasize whatever we want. Fantasies are not actions.
- Someone with a good libido knows the difference between fantasy and reality.
- Someone with a good libido does not act out their fantasies willy-nilly.
- The natural form of libido does not lead to any bad things.
- When someone is out of control and pushes themselves onto others, that is bad behavior. That has nothing to do with libido.
- A good healthy libido that is expressed appropriately is a marvelous thing.
- When we see that in action, we may even be envious.
- We too may wish for that kind of joy and juiciness.

## However, in men, libido is also a *global sense of well-being*:

- It is not just sexual.
- It is the sense of fully being a man.
- It is a feeling of being powerfully engaged in life and effective in the world.
- You have agency in the world.
- People respond to you as an attractive man.
- You are basking in the vitality of full authentic masculinity.

- You feel that in yourself, and the world perceives that in you.

## The decline of sexual desire and male well-being:

- It is surprisingly common in men of any age.
- It is especially common in middle-aged guys.
- It often progresses so slowly that you don't really notice it.
- You may think to yourself: This is just part of getting older.
- You may not realize that you can do something about it.
- And you may have forgotten how very much it matters.

## When libido is lacking:

- With low libido, men have depressed moods.
- And when they are depressed, their libido is low.
- This is a negative feedback loop about depression and libido.
- The men feel flat. Not juicy. Not alive.
- They do not feel like the king of the mountain.
- They do not feel happy.
- They may be irritable and cranky.
- They may be envious of the virile men they see around them.
- They may not dress well or groom well.
- They do not feel attractive. That feeling is painful.
- These feelings are hidden.
- In our society we judge men for being "too sexual."

- And we do not realize how their sexuality is woven into the core of their being.
- Here I am talking about depressed mood. Not severe clinical depression which needs psychiatric care.

## A key insight into men:

- When you think juicy thoughts about sexual topics, it makes you happy. It elevates your mood. It gives you energy. It makes life worth living. It makes the world go around.
- When you do not feel this, then it's hard to get out of bed in the morning. The world exists only in black and white, no color. Life feels flat and dull.

## How to get your libido back:

- Daily Cialis improves male libido—to a varying extent in different men.
- DC improves blood flow and micro perfusion in the pelvis which serves to revitalize that whole area.
- However, testosterone also improves libido quickly and effectively.
- It wakes up the male sexual desire again.
- This is one way how testosterone works well for men who have depressive moods.

## When you have your libido back:

- You feel like King of the Mountain again.
- You feel like you can tackle the world.

- As one of my patients put it: "Life is happening in living color."
- You feel that life is worth living.
- You smile. You feel happy. You feel like a real man.
- You enjoy all the good things the world has to offer, including the visuals of attractive individuals around you.
- I love it when patients say to me: "I forgot how good it feels to feel good."
- The men got back what they used to have.
- They had not realized how much they had lost.
- And the juicy and alive feelings were even better than they remembered.

## Information for women:

We generally think of libido as a feeling, an emotion, a state of being;

Something that exists in the brain and maybe in the heart.

Something that is a part of one's whole being.

## However, in men it is different than in women:

It was surprising to learn this about men:

- Libido is not just in the genitals.
- Libido is not just in the mind.
- Libido is in the body too.
- Libido is in every part of men's being.
- It is *the* key component of a man's well-being.
- Women often do not realize that for men, their libido truly is their life force.

- For many women, life force and libido are experienced separately.
- Men have frequent, strong and physical reminders of their sexual nature by their bodies' obvious reactions.
- Women may have that too —hopefully—however usually not as clearly.
- A man feels it in his physical organ—which is difficult to ignore.
- Women often do not realize how present men's sexual energy is literally in their bodies.
- Women sometimes tend to disparage men's sexuality.
- How did our society make it okay to express this kind of disrespect to other human beings?

## The "dirty old man" thing:

- When young handsome men are visibly in their virile power, we tend to appreciate that.
- Men's nature stays the same as they get older.
- Their bodies may not look as sexy. They may be less cute to look at.
- However, their sexuality still feels the same to them.
- And suddenly we call them "dirty old men"—even if their behavior has not changed.
- Again: Acting out of control and pushing oneself onto others, that is bad behavior. That has nothing to do with libido.
- Even if men behave normally, the way they did when they were younger, we judge them.
- Again: How did our society make it okay to express this kind of disrespect to other human beings?

- Maybe we can create some awareness about this paradox.

## In closing:

- Let's remember to value and support men's libido as an expression of their global well-being.
- Men may use Daily Cialis to support their libido.
- Men may choose to use testosterone for a powerful restoration of their life force.

# Rapid Ejaculation

What is rapid ejaculation?

How can it be improved?

Which methods work best?

Of all the major male sexual problems—erectile dysfunction, delayed orgasm, and rapid ejaculation (RE) —the last one is the most difficult in many ways.

With rapid ejaculation, especially if it is more severe, the problem can be very distressing for a man. And, even though there are approaches to improving it, they are usually complex and take time.

Rapid ejaculation used to be called premature ejaculation. These days actually many of us in the sex positive world call it "coming before he wants to." That is more accurate, but it is a cumbersome phrase.

## So, what is the definition of this sexual problem?

It is a tricky one to define because the range is so very wide. The range is from men who come as early as the first contact of penis with vagina, all the way to men who are basically okay but would like to last longer or have more ejaculatory control.

Diagnosticians have at times tried to define this issue by the length of duration of intercourse. However, who is to say what is the proper or normal length for intercourse? This question, of course, is meaningless because it varies so much from couple to couple, and from one love making session to the next.

"What's normal?" is never a useful question in sex therapy. We want that individual and that couple to have more satisfying sex—in whatever ways they want.

We are *not* aiming for normal sex (like we might aim for a normal blood sugar level). We are aiming for more pleasure and more satisfaction for that individual man and for that individual couple, as they themselves define that.

## More than half of men have experienced RE:

What is important to note is that number of men who come before they want to (or their partner wants them to) is huge. It is or has been an issue to some degree for the majority of men. So, in a way, it can be seen as just a challenge with sex in general. And then again, for the men for whom it is severe, it is not "just a challenge," it is really a difficult problem.

It does not help that many thoughtless jokes and judgements about this issue are prevalent in our society. I cringe when I hear those comments and jokes. I would suggest that you also commit to avoiding them, just like we avoid racial or religious comments.

So, in this chapter, I will focus on approaches for men who feel that they come *much* earlier than they want to.

## Rapid ejaculation can have far-reaching consequences:

- Men can have less confidence in themselves sexually.

- In really severe situations, the men will start to avoid sexual situations because they have been so stressful for them in the past.
- The men often feel that this is difficult to discuss with a new partner.
- The men may waste money and effort on ineffective solutions on the Internet.

## How to improve RE:

For other sexual issues, there are many solutions to try alone or with partner at home. And there are certainly things to try for this issue also. They are mentioned below.

In my opinion, for the more frustrating situations, the most effective solution is to work with a sex therapist.

## How to choose a sex therapist:

Take your choosing process *very* seriously. It is gratifying to me how many truly great sex therapists are out there. And also, it is shocking and terrifying to me how many are ineffective or may even subtly sabotage the work due to their own unseen discomfort. You may need to spend time driving some distance for your sex therapist appointments.

A really great resource for finding a good sex therapist is AASECT: American Association of Sexuality Educators, Counselors, and Therapists: https://www.aasect.org.

Coming before you want to is often treated with a partner. The sex therapist will give instructions to the man and his

partner for the exercises. And these exercises will progress as
the sex therapy progresses.

## What is a sexual surrogate?

If the man is single or if his partner does not want to do the
exercises with him, a sexual surrogate is a really effective
solution. Sexual surrogates have extensive training to work with
clients who have sexual problems. Their work includes talking,
all kinds of touch, and actual sex, including intercourse, if
indicated.

Sexual surrogates only work with a client when there is also a
sex therapist involved. Sexual surrogates can be male and
female, and either can work with men and women. They have
average looks and bodies, just like regular sexual partners do.
They are also trained in ethics and interpersonal dynamics: The
work with them will definitely *not* lead to a relationship.

Sexual surrogates work with all kinds of sexual issues.
However, in my opinion, they are especially useful for rapid
ejaculation.

The International Professional Surrogates Association IPSA is
professional, ethical, and effective. Everyone benefits by knowing
that they exist and what they do:
http://www.surrogatetherapy.org.

IPSA can refer you to a sex therapist who is used to working
with them. In my experience, only a few sex therapists are
experienced in working with surrogates. So, you may wish to
choose your sex therapist with IPSA's recommendations to begin
with.

It can take some effort to contact these sex therapists and sexual surrogates. I don't know why that is, but often it can take repeated contact to do the initial organizing. So, don't take that personally, and don't take it as a reflection of their professional expertise.

Typically, the client works with a surrogate (actual sexual contact) and also with a sex therapist (talking therapy) at the same time. Yes, that is not cheap. But how much is it worth to have a satisfying sex life for the rest of your life? I would encourage you to go ahead and invest in your own sexual pleasure, and in your present and future relationships in this way: This will make a big difference in the quality of your life!

If you are not sure, you can always just talk with the people that you contact via IPSA and AASECT to get more information. You do not need to make a decision right away.

## Working with your own partner:

If a man has a partner who really does want to do the exercises with him, and the dynamics between them are relaxed and positive, then they can try using a book like *Sexual Healing* by Barbara Keesling. Or for greater effectiveness, they can go to a sex therapist together. In that case, the man may not use a sexual surrogate.

## Useful Concepts for RE:

- Definitely good to do: Pelvic muscle control/Kegels.
- Decrease sensation by using a condom.

- The antidepressant medications called SSRI's can help. They all can be effective with Paxil (paroxetine) leading the pack.
- Some touch exercises called *Sensate Focus exercises* can be very useful.
- The purpose of these exercises is to learn to enjoy the touch again, rather than focusing on sexual performance or orgasm.
- These exercises and sensate focus are explained in detail in the *Sexual Healing* book by Barbara Keesling.

## Concepts that are used with some effectiveness:

- Stop/Start technique: Stop movement until the urge to come passes.
- Squeeze technique: Squeezing under the head of the penis until the urge to come passes.
- Testicle tugging: To delay the urge to come.
- Numbing creams inside a condom—not usually a good idea.

## Cialis and Viagra:

- Viagra can lengthen the window from arousal to ejaculation in some men
- Cialis and Daily Cialis can also help lengthen that window.
- When Sexual Performance Anxiety has set in, Cialis and Viagra can help.
- Check out the chapter on Sexual Performance Anxiety too.

## Cialis helps with Rapid Ejaculation:

- Viagra and Levitra also can improve RE. Sometimes one of these three medications will work better that the others for an individual man.
- These medications increase confidence, therefore promoting a more relaxed feeling.
- RE can be associated with some degree of erectile dysfunction because everything gets so complicated from the stress. Cialis and Daily Cialis help with that.
- It can increase the chances that the man can stay erect after ejaculation.
- It can decrease the refractory period. So that the man can have an erection again sooner.
- In a research study, these medications increased overall sexual satisfaction in RE situations.

# Sexual Performance Anxiety

When does sexual performance anxiety come up for *you*?

How would it feel to be really present in your body during sex?

What do you do when you worry about your sexual performance?

## Case Study:

Mark is a handsome divorced man in his mid-fifties who wanted to date more when he started his medical visits with me. He had not had sex in 4 years. Before then, his erections had been unreliable. So, he was anxious about the idea of being on a date where sex might come up.

When he had first become single, he had gone out on some dates. After suffering through several frustrating sexual encounters with no successful erections, he had given up completely on dating. He also had prostate issues with urinary urgency, and frequency. These symptoms also made him shy about being social.

Once on DC, it turned out that he needed a larger dose. When he settled in on that dosage, he noticed some happy effects. He occasionally had morning erections. He also noticed improvement in his bladder symptoms so that it was easier for him to be out on the town.

He did get brave and started to date again. He took it slow and made a point of getting to know a woman before having sex. This strategy helped him feel more connected. With this behavioral learning plus the Daily Cialis, he was delighted to be having fun again with women. He is a changed man!

## Sexual performance anxiety can be very distressing to men:

- They usually do not feel comfortable talking about it.
- So, it becomes a secret that keeps getting worse.
- It can become more severe with repeated upsetting experiences.
- It can be so debilitating that the man completely avoids potentially sexual situations, like dating.
- Then he is caught in a negative spiral.
- Cialis and Viagra are very effective in this situation.
- There are also many non-medical ways to improve it.
- These non-medical ideas work best in conjunction with the ED medications.

## Sexual performance anxiety can detract from your sexual experience, causing you to:

- Focus more on the performance than your own pleasure, and
- Therefore feel less pleasure.
- Focus more on your performance than feeling your partner, and
- Therefore feel less connected.
- Rush things along to use an erection as soon as it appears.

- Rush things along to have an ejaculation to make sure that happens.
- Move along a standard script rather than following your desire in the moment.
- Not feel relaxed.
- Not feel trust and closeness with your partner, and
- As a result of all that, have decreased sexual function in different ways.

This whole situation is a double-edged sword because it really does matter whether a man cares about the quality of his love making for his partner's benefit. When a man with ED issues does not make the effort to learn about the skills and the medications to optimize his function, that impacts his partner too. When a man or woman does not make the effort to keep learning more sexual skills, the partner will not have as much fun.

## Cialis and Viagra work really well for sexual performance anxiety:

- He can relax and have fun again.
- He gets a break from the worrying.
- The man can get his confidence back.
- He feels like a man again.
- On demand Cialis works well for this purpose.
- If he is in a relationship or in a situation where he might want to have sex anytime, then Daily Cialis can be a great solution.
- Once he feels more comfortable, he can decrease dosage or even stop it, if he does not have ED.

## How to use Cialis and Viagra for sexual performance anxiety?

- When a man feels anxiety about an upcoming sexual situation because he has had distressing experiences with ED in the past, then he is stuck in a vicious cycle.
- Taking Cialis or Daily Cialis will make a big difference in breaking that pattern.
- Then, over time, the man will regain confidence that sex can indeed be pleasant for him.
- If the sexual occasions are fairly frequent or spontaneous, DC is a good plan.
- If the sexual occasions are rare, he may wish to use on-demand Viagra or Cialis.
- He should try both of them at home by himself to become familiar with them.
- It works best for him to take the ED medications consistently until he really feels comfortable.
- It is important to reinforce the pleasure and fun part of each sexual experience.
- If he uses the pills only intermittently, there is the risk that the performance anxiety will be reinforced by unpleasant experiences. We do not want that.

## Being sexually confident in different settings:

- Some men usually do not have ED but they want some reassurance in certain settings.
- For example, it could be the first time with a new partner or sex in a distracting setting.
- They may take Viagra or Cialis for that occasion.

- They may find that it works like Dumbo's feather in the Disney movie: They know that it is on board (perhaps they have a stuffy nose to prove it) so they can relax.
- And, of course, being relaxed is a good thing for better erections.
- When a man takes Daily Cialis, then he is already covered for these occasional situations.
- Some men find though, that their usual dose of Daily Cialis is not enough for these more challenging situations.
- In those cases, some of them may choose to take a higher dose of Cialis that day.
- You can ask your doctor about taking a higher dose of Cialis at certain times.

## How to approach sexual performance anxiety:

A sexual encounter is a mix of inward and outward experiences. You have your own sensations and feelings inside you. And also, you are aware of your appearance and your actions as seen by your partner. Ideally there is a balance between those two factors so that you enjoy yourself and are relaxed, and also you pay attention to your impact on your partner. Ideally sex is a pleasurable experience and an intimate connection, not a performance.

Women often have their own issues, usually with focusing too much on how they think they look. They may focus more on holding in their stomach than on the yummy sensations in their bodies. They may avoid certain sexual positions, which they actually enjoy, because they feel their breasts look too droopy or their butt looks too big. That is a pity, isn't it? They would have so much more fun just focusing on the pleasures they are feeling.

However similar issues can come up for men: They often worry about how their partner perceives their sexual performance, to the point of losing the awareness of their delicious sensations. They may have a set of high expectations for themselves. They may have a list of goals to achieve.

They feel the pressure to get and maintain an erection right on cue. And then they feel that they need to have an ejaculatory orgasm when the time is right for the woman: Not too early, not too late. They may feel uncomfortable if they cannot or do not wish to have an ejaculation at that time. Men fake orgasms too.

Ideally both partners continually move back and forth along the spectrum of enjoying the sensations in their own bodies, enjoying their partner's body, and focusing on their partner's pleasure. Sexual performance anxiety severely limits the scope of that spectrum: The experience becomes all about measuring up to some external theoretical construct.

To add to the unhappy mix, sometimes the sexual performance anxiety expresses itself via situational erectile dysfunction. This can even happen in men who usually do not have ED issues. Once a man has had the experience of sexual performance anxiety combined with erection problems, then the fear of a repeat unhappy experience can start a negative feedback loop. This is when the suggestions below—about what to do beforehand and in the moment—combined with the judicious use of erection meds can help to create a positive feedback loop again. That way the man can regain his confidence. And with the confidence he will have the relaxation and fun of anxiety-free sexual play.

Porn is a complex issue, and in general is not as bad as it is made out to be. However, one of the risks of watching porn is internalizing the movie sequences—and the action sequences—to some extent. Even though we don't do a car chase on the streets of San Francisco after watching a Steve McQueen movie, we do have sex after watching porn. And even though men as well as women theoretically know that their own experience is not a movie, there can be some subtle—and not so subtle "bad" learning of how to do sex "right." This is one way that men sometimes feel pressure to perform.

## What to do about sexual performance anxiety ahead of time:

- Talk with your partner about the performance anxiety feelings.

- Keep talking with your partner about what you both like to do and to receive during sensual and sexual play—that makes for great dinner and driving conversations.

- Talk about fantasies: Both the fantasy-fantasies that you do not expect to act out and the fantasies that could be incorporated into a love making session.

- Talk about what you know that you enjoy. And things you would enjoy trying.

- Ask your partner. Observe your partner. To keep learning more about what they like.

- How can you best remember what your partner does (and does not) like? Maybe even take notes?

## What to do when sexual performance anxiety comes up during sex play:

- Slow *way* down: breathe, smile, cuddle, caress.

- Make time for nonsexual touch—enjoy the sensuality.

- Don't separate "foreplay" and "real sex." Mix it up. Go back and forth.

- Encourage your partner to give you touch and caresses by making happy noises, responding with your body, speaking brief words of gratitude.

- Express yourself: Make little requests, speak appreciations and affections.

- Truly enjoy your partner: How they feel, how they smell, how they taste, how they move.

- Truly enjoy your own body: Feel the sensations, move in response to them.

- Keep focusing on enjoying *all* your senses.

- Take responsibility for your own orgasm. And encourage your partner to do that too.

- Keep exploring—for both of you—having orgasms in different ways.

- Play with tantra ideas: Sex can start anywhere, go anywhere, pause anytime.

- Alcohol and pot can make things worse. Best used lightly.

- Use positive self-talk both inside yourself and out loud to your partner: Speak the yummy things that you are feeling emotionally and physically in the moment.

## The positive outlook:

- Focus on fun and pleasure first—for both partners!

- Continually make an effort to become a better lover.

- Improve and maintain sexual function with available tools.

- Use ED medications the way you find them most useful.

- Ease up on yourself about rigid performance standards.

- Focus on touch and pleasure first—and always!

# Dating and Daily Cialis

How would you feel with more sexual confidence while dating?

What if you are a man with some ED issues, and you want to date?

When have you been concerned about your sexual performance with a new partner?

## Case study:

Al is a 62-year-old all-around good guy who is liked by everyone. His appearance is average, and his body could use a little more exercise. He is happy except for his fear of dating.

He has not had sex in a while. And at that time, he had problems getting erections. He is worried that if he dates again, he will find someone who wants to have sex, but he will not be able to have an erection. This worry makes him anxious on his dates, and so he does not have fun.

He also has some issues with needing to go to the bathroom often and has to hurry to get there. This also makes dates and other outings less fun and more anxiety producing for him.

He was very curious when I talked with him about the concept of Daily Cialis for the sexual issue as well as the bladder and prostate problem. He was very ready to get started. As always, we worked until we found the optimal dose for him.

When he was taking this effective dose, he could tell that his sexuality was bubbling again because he was back to occasional morning erections. He also noted that his urination problems improved.

Now he loves to go on dates. And when he and his date decide to have sex, he feels ready and confident. Now he enjoys himself on dates!

When a man is in a dating situation, some issues are similar to a long-term relationship situation. And some issues are different.

When you are on a first date with a woman, you may have mixed feelings about the possibility of sex. Perhaps you are very attracted to her and want to make a good impression. You may feel pressure to perform, and you may be worried how that will go. And, at the same time, you may also wish for sex. You may be excited by the thought of sex with her.

Perhaps you have not had sex in a while. Perhaps there have been some instances in the past where the erections were not optimal. Basically, all men have had those experiences. Maybe you have even had more serious ED issues.

## Here are important pointers:

- Do not drink any alcohol. (Or maybe just a half a standard drink, absolutely no more.) At home people tend to make drinks bigger than at a bar or restaurant, so be careful.
- Have sex before dinner, not after. A full stomach does not improve things for either of you.

## Moving into erotic connection:

- Do not rush into sex with this new woman. Over the course of the first date or the first dates, do a lot of nonsexual touching, cuddling and other body contact to get you two connected. This will get you both more comfortable.

- Also do different things together on your dates: Share each other's hobbies. Get outdoors. Be social with friends. That way you both will feel more familiar with each other. Touch and sex will flow more naturally.

- Some women are raring to get to the sex, others not so much. Talk about this with her. She will be thrilled that you care enough to talk.

- It is okay if you do not want to rush into sex. Just tell her that you like to know her better before you get to sex.

- However, don't wait too long if she wants sex. Do not let too many dates go by. Otherwise she may conclude that you cannot or will not have sex. Also, your and her anxiety will go up if you wait too long. Sometimes it is good to just dive right in and create that connection.

- Ask her: What do you like when you make love? What are your favorite things? What bothers you during sex? What is your sexuality like? What is her favorite lube? Then buy that lube.

- And be prepared to share some information about yourself.

- You will make better impression if you say that you like to give and receive oral sex. It does not sound good when a guy comes on strongly about needing to receive oral sex.

## How do you choose whom to date?

- This is extremely important. Many men with less dating experience have not learned this yet: If you date normal, regular women you will be more relaxed and have way more fun than if you go for the most beautiful and most popular gals.
- You may feel intimidated by the glamorous women. Therefore, you will not be your authentic self and then not enjoy yourself as much.

## Using Cialis optimally:

- While dating, take your Cialis or Daily Cialis as you normally do.
- Test drive the medication by yourself at home to figure out your optimal dose.

## Key pointers about condoms:

- Condoms can make an ED situation more difficult.
- Consider trying the female condom. It has more room inside. Therefore, it gives you more sensation.
- You can buy the female condom online, and get instructions for it online.
- Make the effort to try different kinds of condoms so that you find your favorite one. Find the size that works for you and does not strangle you.
- Often the condoms with more space at the tip will give you more sensation, which is good.
- Don't bother with the ribbed and other fancy condoms.

- It's more important to try different kinds and different shapes that to find what *you* like best.
- Have some lube handy in case she does not have any.
- I think the Pjur Original silicone lube in the black bottle is very good. You can buy it online.
- Have the condom ready: Have it within arm's reach. Risk the 50 cents and tear open the package beforehand. Take the condom out, put it on top of the wrapper, and remember which side is up.
- You want to put the condom on quickly to keep the sexual energy flowing for you both and to preserve the erection.

## Safer Sex:

- You will want to talk about your safer sex situation with each other. The Planned Parenthood website and the San Francisco Sex Information website are good resources. Don't wait to educate yourself: Read that now.
- Then you will decide together whether to use condoms.
- Typically, in a sexual encounter that is spontaneous and with an unfamiliar partner, you will use condoms.

## If you are having sex and the erection is not happening:

- Take a break from attempts at intercourse. Instead just give her oral sex while you stimulate yourself.
- Take a break from sex completely. Do some back massage. Maybe even go for a walk and then come back and play again.
- It is a turnoff for women when the man gets frantic when there is no erection and wants more and more oral sex or

stimulation by her hand—with no results. Better to take a break and reassess.

- Remember that, even with Cialis, the body needs sexual stimulation for the penis to get hard. If you just sit around watch the ball game and wait for the erection to happen—it won't. The stimulation can be by her or by yourself.

- You may wish to talk with your doctor about possibly using more Cialis on days with dates.

## And do remember the secret recipe:

- You'd be surprised how many men don't do this—and it costs them!

- The *most* effective skill of all: listen to her in a way that feeds her!

- Sweet and connected conversation creates intimacy that is quite sexy:

  o   1) Ask her about her day,

  o   2) listen to the answer, and

  o   3) then ask another question related to what she just said.

- After every two or three sets of questions like that, share something *intimate and personal* about yourself to prevent the interview vibe. You may wish to think of those shares ahead of time, before going into a social setting, because it can be hard to think on the spot.

- Being listened to and shared with makes a woman feel appreciated and cared for.

- Practice this every day in any and all social settings. It is more difficult to do than one thinks. You may think that you are doing it—but actually she is the one who is getting you to talk—which is not good! It also is *way* more important than most men realize. If you only learn one skill from this entire book, this skill will make the most difference in your life and relationships!

Remember: The point of dating is for both you and her to have fun and to enjoy the connection! So, have a good time!

# Delayed Ejaculation — Difficult for the Man to Come

## Case Study:

James was 51 years old and married. He had been a patient in my office for a few years, and was treated, successfully, for low libido. He responded well to testosterone and was glad to have his sexual desire back.

He enjoys intercourse and his ejaculatory orgasms. So, he was distressed when he found that it was getting more difficult for him to reach orgasm. This is called Delayed Ejaculation (DE). He was very worried. He was also having some ED issues.

So I started him on Daily Cialis for the erection problem. DC does not always fix DE but it can sometimes help. And we also talked about things to do during sex to improve his orgasms.

Much to his delight and relief, the Daily Cialis not only fixed his erection problems but also his Delayed Orgasm. He is back to enjoying his regular orgasms. He is a happy man again!

## Working around Delayed Orgasm:

As men get into middle age and beyond, a surprisingly high number start to have trouble reaching their ejaculatory orgasm. Whereas they used to take their orgasm for granted, suddenly they find that it has become an elusive pleasure.

It may take a lot more effort and time to get to orgasm. Or it may be the case that it still works fine with masturbation but not with intercourse. Typically, the orgasm with intercourse is the first thing to go.

Some men, who used to worry that their orgasm would happen too soon, now find that that it takes a lot of effort to orgasm. Or maybe it hardly happens at all.

Men react very differently to this situation of difficulty reaching orgasm. Some men like to make love for long periods of time. And they like to be ready for sex anytime without the refractory period. They find that they have better energy and desire for sex if they don't come too often. So they do not consider delayed ejaculation a major problem.

Some men like to experiment with having additional orgasms that are non-ejaculatory. They are more full-body focused or more of an energy peak. The concept of male multiple orgasm includes these kinds of orgasms. This is why I specifically use the term ejaculatory orgasms: To differentiate that kind of orgasm from other kinds of orgasm.

One solution is to find what does work to produce the ejaculatory orgasm: Their own or their partner's hands. Perhaps oral sex also works better than intercourse. A combination of oral and manual stimulation can work very well.

So these men are okay with not having an orgasm every time. They realize that, as they get older, their sexuality is likely to change and decrease in function in some ways. Many men feel that, "If I have any kind of sexual problem, this is a good one to have."

## When Delayed Ejaculation is a Problem:

Some men are extremely upset about the loss of the easy and frequent ejaculatory orgasm. They really love the routine of sexual intercourse culminating in an orgasm. When this decreases or becomes more difficult, they keenly feel the loss, and they worry about their sexual pleasure in the future.

For health professionals like me who talk with men about their sexual issues, delayed ejaculation can be especially frustrating. There is usually no straightforward solution.

And this situation can be exacerbated by the use of a condom which cuts down on the sensation. If a condom is needed, it can help to use a female condom. If you search for "female condom" online, you will see how to buy the current version and how to use them. Be sure to put lube inside the female condom for more sensation.

Or a man can try different types of male condoms to see which ones give him the most sensation. The male condoms with a bigger tip, which have more space for the head of the penis, often work better.

## Sometimes there can be surprising solutions:

The lucky patient in the case study got his orgasms back. This has happened occasionally in my practice but not routinely.

Research has shown repeatedly that both intermittent Cialis and Daily Cialis can significantly improve orgasmic dysfunction and ejaculatory dysfunction in men of all ages.

It does not make sense that DC would help both with delayed ejaculation and with rapid ejaculation (coming before he wants to). However, the fact is that it can help with both of these situations even though they seem to be opposing problems. It is my hypothesis that DC works by normalizing the function of the ejaculatory orgasm.

If delayed ejaculation is an issue for you, you might try Daily Cialis and observe the results.

# The Last Taboo: Prostate Health

- Why is prostate health the key to youthful vigor?
- How can you fight for your prostate wellness?
- Which bladder problems are affecting you now?
- A healthy prostate is key to feeling young and masculine.
- However, have you noticed that no one talks about prostate health?
- It is the last taboo, the last unspeakable thing.
- And yet, this important gland holds the key to your present and future masculine health.

The poor prostate gland clearly has a public relations problem: Young guys really don't want to think about it. And for older guys it is nothing but trouble. Have you noticed: Talk about prostate cancer is everywhere. But no one ever talks about prostate health and well-being.

Be sure and pronounce the word correctly: There is only one R in it. You say "pro" as in "I'm pro prostate health." And then "state" as in "state of health."

Say: "Pro-state." It is amazing how much trouble people have with this word. Maybe it reflects the ambivalent feelings people have about this gland!

## Prostate and Bladder Problems:

Prostate symptoms are caused by Benign Prostatic Hypertrophy (BPH) which is an enlarged prostate. BPH is not cancer.

## Bladder symptoms due to BPH:

- Urgent need to urinate.
- Difficulty starting the stream.
- Weak flow. It takes a long time.
- Dribbling afterwards.
- Feeling of incomplete emptying.
- Needing to go again soon.
- Pain or strange sensations before and during urination.
- Need to urinate very frequently
  - o Daytime: It is inconvenient.
  - o Nighttime: It disturbs sleep (for the partner too).
  - o Both partners are sleep deprived and unhappy.

These bladder symptoms are called *Lower Urinary Tract Symptoms* (LUTS). They are extremely common in men in their fifties and older. They will steadily get worse over time and will seriously affect your quality of life.

When you observe middle-aged and older men around you, you will notice that many of them go to the bathroom often. And they stay in there for quite a while. This is why some of them choose to sit down to urinate: Because it takes so long that they get tired of standing. These concerns plus the erection problems make a man—and his partner—feel old.

Statistics say that about half of older men are affected. My observation, both in my practice and in everyday life, is that it is much more prevalent than that. My observation is that almost all men who are middle-aged or older have this problem to some degree.

The prostate problems will not get better nor go away on their own. They just get worse. If you have some symptoms now, how will you be in ten years? In twenty years? Don't let that happen.

## Prostate and Bladder Solution:

- Daily Cialis reliably reduces the symptoms of BPH.
- This treatment for prevention and treatment of prostate symptoms is safe, easy, and effective.
- Daily Cialis is officially approved by the FDA for BPH.
- It is the only medication that treats both ED and BPH.
- Cialis helps LUTS by relaxing the smooth muscle in the prostate and bladder.
- This effect also increases blood circulation in the prostate. Increased circulation is good for the tissues.
- Men like Daily Cialis because their urination is more normal which, in turn, makes them feel younger and more vital.
- Men like DC also because it also turns back the clock on erectile function.
- Men have fewer trips to the bathroom at night so they (and their partners) sleep better and feel more rested.
- If you start Daily Cialis now, you can be your optimal masculine self now.
- And you will also be your best optimal self in 10 and 20 years.

## Talk with your doctor:

- If you are taking other prostate medications, you need to let your doctor know. You may need to start Cialis at lower dose to minimize reactions.

- Some BPH medications can worsen ED. They are called *alpha blockers*. Flomax (tamsulosin) is a well-known medication in this category.

- Be sure to consult your doctor closely on all these matters to get the best results with the most safety.

# Benefits of Testosterone

What are your levels of sexual confidence and sexual desire right now?

How are your moods these days?

What is Hormonophobia?

## Case Study:

Joseph is in his fifties. He works in a large company where he would like to get ahead. He came to me with the problem that he had lost his goal-oriented focus and his competitive spirit. He was also trying to fight off some extra pounds and was not getting to the gym as much as he would like.

His decreased erections prevented him and his wife from fully enjoying their sex life. He and his wife also did not like waiting for the erection pill to kick in, each time they wanted sex. They really wanted to be able to have spontaneous sex.

Once he was started on his combination of DC and testosterone, they were thrilled to be able to make love again anytime, on the spur of the moment. Joseph felt that he was on top of his game in his company. He was able to stick with his goals of eating less. He also had plenty of energy at the gym.

He said, "Thank you for giving me my life back!"

She told him to tell me, "Thank you for giving me my husband back!"

Gentlemen: Here is another tool for your tool box. This one definitely is a power tool. Every man needs this information to know the possibilities that are available to him, anytime he chooses.

Daily Cialis is one of the two main pillars to high-powered sexual and global well-being in middle age. The other pillar is testosterone (T).

DC and T together are the dynamic duo! They create a synergy for good sexual function plus strong libido and positive moods. They can give you the Best Sex Ever!

Most people don't know the truth about T: It is a bioidentical hormone that has a many positive effects in body, emotions, and mind.

## In this chapter:

- You will get an overview of:
- The symptoms of low testosterone.
- The benefits of T therapy.
- The myths.
- The risks and cautions.
- What T therapy looks like.
- Double Trouble: The misery of simultaneous Menopause and Andropause.
- Be sure to read about Hormonophobia at the end of the chapter.

## Symptoms of low T:

Often a wife or partner will see these symptoms more clearly than the man himself:

- Low sexual desire
- Irritable or cranky moods
- Less physical endurance
- Workouts are less effective
- Decreased muscle mass
- Takes longer to recharge after exertion
- Depressive moods
- Anxious or nervous moods
- Lack of focus or goal orientation or drive
- Overwhelm or feeling that life is hard
- Lack of grooming
- Unsatisfying orgasms
- Lack of confidence
- Lack of generosity
- Angry moods
- Osteoporosis
- Brain fog
- Indecisiveness
- Fatigue, lack of energy
- Diminished enthusiasm for life

## Double Trouble:

Andropause (in men) together with menopause (in women).

You can see how it could be really hard on a relationship:

- The long time of being in the marriage is taking its toll. You are way past the honeymoon stage.
- She is cranky and has low sexual desire. Life feels unmanageable to her.
- He is irritable. He feels like his masculinity is decreasing, and typically does not have anyone to talk with about this.
- Both are not having fun. They are not feeling happy.
- It is easy to blame these feelings on the relationship and on the partner.
- They both do not realize that these problems can be improved—in ways that are safe, straightforward, and scientific.
- What would it be to try hormone therapy for both partners before thinking about divorce?
- Hormone therapy for even one of the partners can help the relationship.
- In my practice there has been more than one divorce prevented by hormone therapy.
- The funny thing: When you are on hormones and feel better, you forget how miserable it feels to be miserable. Feeling good is the new normal.
- The corollary: When you are not on hormones, you don't realize that your misery is largely physiological, not psychological.
- It's so great to hear this in my practice, "I forgot how good it feels to feel good!"

## Benefits of T therapy:

- The libido and mood benefits can happen surprisingly quickly: Sometimes in just a few days.
- Positive mood.
- Improved libido and sexual desire.
- Increase in endurance, strength, and exercise capacity.
- Stronger bones. Osteoporosis is a serious issue for men too.
- Better brain function.
- Increase in muscle mass, reduction in body fat.
- Workouts have greater effect.
- More energy.
- More assertiveness and confidence.
- Helps with ED, especially over the long-term.
- Greater vigor and vitality.
- More drive, more focus.
- More vision, more goal oriented.
- Men with high T levels live longer, per recent research.
- Improvements in high BMI, larger waist circumference, diabetes, high cholesterol, and heart disease.
- For men with depressive moods, it can be worthwhile to consider T before considering antidepressants. You need to consult with an experienced doctor about that specific situation.
- T has men be out on the court playing, rather than sitting on the sidelines watching—literally as well as figuratively.

## Lack of libido is connected to depressive moods in men:

For many men, depressive symptoms are combined with lack of libido. One major benefit of T—that can happen quite quickly—is increased libido or sexual desire.

When men do not feel juicy and sexual, they do not feel alive. Being sexually confident gives men that feeling of male life force that they need. Women in our culture do not usually realize how much men need that sexual presence to feel on top of the world.

Unfortunately, men are often criticized for their interest in sex when actually, their sexuality is closely tied up with their entire being. In order to feel happy and masculine they need to feel the occasional stirring in their loins. And with T they can have those feelings back.

## How to manage T therapy:
- These benefits vary by individuals, by how low their levels were to begin with, and by how optimal their T doses are.
- Testosterone should be given only when needed, in appropriate amounts, and with careful supervision.
- It may take some focus and time to get the T level optimal for *you*.
- T is a complex substance and needs to be monitored by an experienced health practitioner to get the best results.

## Risks:

- An occasional pimple, usually only at the beginning of T therapy.
- Temporary reduction of sperm count, which is an issue only if there are plans for pregnancy.
- In rare cases: A man will increase his red blood cells enough that he needs to donate blood. This is monitored and corrected by the doctor.

## While you are on T therapy:

- Using T is actually simple and easy: You just use T cream on your skin every morning.
- Another option is injectable T. That works well too.
- It is important to be monitored by someone who really understands T therapy as well as male physiology and sexuality.
- Monitoring includes labs as well as clinical medical visits for optimal results.
- To get the best results the man has to come in for visits often enough so that the dosages and applications are finely tuned. Not just "good enough."

## How T therapy works:

- The positive results begin somewhere between 10 minutes and 10 days.
- This testosterone is completely bioidentical. It is the exact same molecule that your own body makes.
- The body never gets addicted to T. You can always decrease it or stop it at any time without adverse effects.

- The body never becomes habituated. You will never need more to get the same effect.
- So there is no point in "saving" T therapy for later. You might as well feel better now.
- It can be useful to do a trial: Use T for 1 to 3 months to see the difference for yourself. Then stay with it, or not. This experiment works best if you get up to your optimal level.

## Dispelling Myths and Fears:

- T does not cause prostate cancer.
- T does not cause heart disease.
- T does not cause high blood pressure.
- T does not cause liver problems.
- T does not cause antisocial behavior.
- T does not increase BPH (enlarged prostate).
- T does not cause aggressiveness in therapeutic doses.
- T does not cause you to get huge and muscle-bound in therapeutic doses.
- Check on Dr. Abraham Morgentaler's websites for more details on these topics.

There are some misconceptions about T in the general public and even among doctors. The fact is—and it has been proven many times now—that testosterone does not cause prostate cancer. In fact, prostate cancer occurs in men when their testosterone levels drop. So, it has been hypothesized that the drop in testosterone may be part of the cause of prostate cancer.

Contrary to another myth, T does not cause BPH symptoms to worsen. In fact, BPH symptoms usually get better with T on board.

## Can you increase your testosterone level without taking testosterone?

- Can certain foods, exercise, or supplements increase T?

- No, those things do not ever reliably work. You'd likely be wasting your time and money. If you have symptoms of low T, just go to the doctor and get the real thing.

## Resistance to taking testosterone:

- There can be fear of the "taking the easy way out."
- T has a mixed reputation, since some men take too much and for questionable reasons.
- Hormonophobia—more on that below.

## The Dynamic Duo for Best Sex Ever:

T is not a magic solution for everything: It does not really fix erection issues. However, T in combination with DC provides a synergy that puts men On Top of His Game. He just feels like his best and most confident self.

That way feels natural and uncontrived, because it is! DC and T really are just supporting his own natural and innate function and optimizing it. They do not take over his body or mind. They just add a little "oomph" to what he already has.

## Don't give in to hormonophobia!

*Hormonophobia* is a witty term coined by Dr. Abraham Morgentaler. His article, by the same name, is on his website and on PubMed. Also, do read his fascinating book about testosterone.

This is the Conclusion of Dr. Morgentaler's "Hormonophobia" article:

> "The use of weak studies as proof of danger indicates that cultural (i.e., nonscientific) forces are at play. Negative media stories touting T's risks appear fueled by antipharma sentiment, anger against aggressive marketing, and antisexuality. This stance is best described as "hormonophobia." As history shows, evidence alone may be insufficient to alter a public narrative. The true outrage is that social forces and hysteria have combined to deprive men of a useful treatment without regard for medical science."

## Want more information?

When searching for information, be careful in choosing your source. So much stuff online is incorrect, alarmist, and not science-based.

These resources are useful:

- Dr. Abraham Morgentaler: YouTube videos, his *Testosterone* book, and his website
- Dr. Thierry Hertoghe: YouTube videos and his *Hormone Solutions* book

# Can You Take Supplements Instead?

What is more natural, supplements or Cialis?

Which is more effective and less costly, supplements or Cialis?

Why is Daily Cialis better for you than supplements?

## The facts are:

- Cialis is an extremely effective medication.
- It has an astoundingly good safety profile.
- It has many nonsexual health benefits.
- The sexual and nonsexual benefits have been proven by scientific studies.

## Don't believe these common myths:

- Many people believe that herbs and supplements are "better for you" than Cialis.
- They believe that supplements are more natural than prescription medications.
- They feel strongly that "natural" is always better.
- People often are seduced by some really amazing supplement.
- They are impressed by the impressive words in the ads.
- They feel safer taking a supplement.
- They are fearful about taking a prescription medication.
- They worry that they will need to "detox" after taking prescription medication.

- They worry that the medication will stress their body or their liver.
- They worry that if they take a medication, they will have dreaded mysterious consequences in the distant future.
- They keep hoping to find an herb that will have the same effect.
- They have a subconscious feeling that there is some supplement out there that will give them a miracle.

## How are supplements, vitamins, and herbs different than prescription medications?

- The fact is that we take many different kinds of substances into our bodies every day.
- Some substances we call "food," some we call "herbs" or "vitamins," some we call "supplements."
- Some substances we call "medicines."
- Medicines can be over-the-counter which means no prescription is needed.
- Medicines can also be by prescription—which means that a doctor needs to evaluate your situation.
- There is no inherent difference between over-the-counter and prescription medications.
- Sometimes medicines get switched from prescription to over-the-counter.
- However, medications that are riskier or more prone to abuse will likely be by prescription.
- There is a move to make Cialis an over-the-counter medication in England.
- Many medications come from herbs: Aspirin from birch bark, metformin from French lilac.

- Herbs are usually non-prescription.
- That does not mean that they are automatically safe for anyone at any dose.
- So, can you see that you need to evaluate any substance carefully on its own merits?
- You cannot draw conclusions from its category.

## What I tell my patients about supplements:

- It's okay to take supplements, just be conscious and careful.
- With supplements, be realistic about how effective they are likely to be.
- Be aware of the placebo effect.
- If a friend is all excited about the newest miracle supplement, ask them to give you a report in six months. Usually, by then, they will have lost interest. Or, in the rare cases where it is proving itself, you will get more useful information.
- If you enjoy taking supplements:
  - Take them when you are excited about them. Use the placebo effect consciously for your own benefit.
  - Don't get married to them.
  - Stop taking them when you lose interest, or a different supplement interests you more.
  - Watch your cost: It is easy to spend a lot of money on those bottles of pills.

## My patients also ask:

- "Doc, what if I eat the perfect diet, and exercise perfectly, and meditate, and take really good supplements, then can I do without the prescription medications?"
- "Will other health practices make it so Cialis is not needed?"

## What I tell my patients:

- You can torture yourself trying to do everything perfectly, and still be disappointed.
- Or you can just take the Cialis and get significant results.

It is good for you to have good health habits but don't get obsessed or extreme about them.

It is more important to enjoy life!

These things do matter but do not torture yourself with the quest for perfection:

- No need for a Perfect diet, as long as your diet is pretty good.
- No need for Perfect exercise and fitness, as long as you move your body every day.
- No need for Perfect meditation, as long as you have some peace and quiet in your life.
- No need to detox when taking Cialis. Your body metabolizes it perfectly already.
- Allow yourself to be a human being. We are not perfect and that is okay.

## Is there a little Puritanism inside us?

- Do you think that it is not really okay to pay attention to a good sex life?
- Do you think that this quest is shallow and not worthwhile?
- Do you secretly worry that if you have too much fun now —such as taking Daily Cialis now for your Best Sex Ever— you will have to pay for it later?
- Become conscious of these thoughts and feelings and do not let them run your life!

## Question Authority, including your own!

- Question the assumptions of your social group.
- Peer pressure can apply to adults too.
- Question your own beliefs and assumptions.
- Keep examining your own beliefs.
- Do they still serve you?
- Do they hold up against good scientific research?
- Stand up for your own well-being. Inform yourself.

# For Your Best Sex Ever: Avoid These Pitfalls

What keeps *you* from having Best Sex Ever?

How are *you* sabotaging your Best Sex Ever?

When will *you* make the effort for Best Sex Ever?

## Case Study:

Peter is in his 50's and has had lifelong issues with depressive moods and now has decreased erections. He had taken antidepressants but did not like their impact with weight gain and decreased sexual desire. He felt stuck for several years. He could not find ways to improve the situation. If any possible solution cropped up, he would find reasons for not taking action.

Finally, he heard about my practice, and became my patient. He was very skeptical but that never bothers me because my treatment speaks for itself. After much discussion and explanation—plus his own research in books and on YouTube, mostly by Dr. Abraham Morgentaler—I started him on Daily Cialis and testosterone. Cialis has an antidepressant effect in addition to the sexual benefits. Testosterone consistently and significantly improves moods in men. Testosterone also helps you set goals and take action. Within a week he was feeling more upbeat and positive. He was also already having reliable erections again, that were way better than he had expected.

He told me: "I had forgotten how good it feels to feel good!"

## What are *your* obstacles?

You want Best Sex Ever, right?

You are ready for it.

You feel that you are trying really hard.

But you are not having Best Sex Ever.

## So many patients thank me

- quite frequently
- for having the best sex of their lives
- at midlife and older
- at an age when they were expecting not to have sex at all.

## I now believe that it's possible for absolutely anyone to have their Best Sex Ever

- Or at least have better sex than now,
- *If* they are willing to do what it takes.
- *If* they are willing to put in the work.
- Those things are practical things, and mental and emotional things.
- These things might not be easy.
- Or you might not know about them yet.
- If they were obvious or easy, you would have done it already.

## So, are you ready and willing?

- To identify your obstacles?

- To do the work?
- Even if it is not easy.

## Look at the lists below.

- Make your own lists in your journal or in your electronic device:
    - o What are the things you need to tackle?
    - o Below are the major common issues.
    - o Some pitfalls are practical in nature.
    - o Some pitfalls are mental and emotional in nature.
- Please do also look through the rest of this book for more information.

## Avoid these pitfalls:

## The practical pitfalls:

- Hesitation and procrastination about trying Daily Cialis: having vague fears, not gathering information, and not taking action.
- Did you know that being indecisive is a sign of low testosterone or T? So, when a man just cannot decide whether to try Daily Cialis (DC) or testosterone, that could mean that he is indeed low in T.
- Not taking enough DC to get good results.
- Not reading this book all the way through to get complete information.
- Not making the effort to learn about sex, about your partner, about your own sexuality.

- Not going for your own and your partner's erotic requests, dreams, and wishes.
- Not finding a doctor to collaborate with you on this project.

## The not-taking-action pitfall:

This is a huge pitfall that I see all the time professionally and socially.

- People postpone their dreams until it is too late.
- Don't wait!
- Do it now. Start today!
- Take a first step today. Then identify the next step.
- It's okay for each step to be tiny.
- Just keep taking the tiny steps.
- Look around, then you will see it too: People have a dream. And they postpone it for all sorts of very good reasons. And then they die. Or their partner dies. Or they, or their partner, become ill or disabled.
- One of my sons told me this story:

    A couple bought a beautiful sail boat with the dream of sailing around together. Life got busy with the usual obligations, so they kept postponing it. Then the wife fell ill, and now they will never be able to do it.

    So, the sad husband wants to sell the boat to someone (like my son and his friends) who will actually use it and enjoy it—like the couple never got to do.

- This important lesson holds for life goals as well as sexual pleasure and exploration.

## The resistance pitfall:

- Not dealing with the normal resistance that we all feel.
- Barbara Sher in Lesson 6 of *Live the Life You Love* tells you how to deal with resistance that you did not even know you had.
- You thought it was just lack of time, lack of money or laziness. No one else says it as well as she does. No one else's methods are as easy and work as amazingly well as hers.
- She also talks about that in her amazing audio program *Dare to Live Your Dream* in the section about Resistance Rescue.

## The money pitfall:

- People often will not spend the money to follow their dreams, the erotic ones and the other ones.
- They may feel guilty spending money to have fun.
- This strategy is *not* running out and spending money willy-nilly on whatever crosses your path.
- You need to think with integrity and precision: What will bring you the most good in the long run?
- This strategy is being true to our real dreams and desires, on a deeper level.
- One way to tell the difference between the two:
    - o The shallow desire will be gone by tomorrow.
    - o The deep and authentic desire will continue to come up in your thoughts.

- You can often get 80 percent of what you want with 20 percent of the money if you think creatively and positively.
- If you are not sure how much money you can spend, hire a good financial advisor.
- Be sure to pick someone who understands emotional needs as well as financial needs.

## The all-or-nothing pitfall:

Spend the money and time now to give yourself some of the *touchstones* of your dreams. *Touchstone* is a term Barbara Sher uses; it is taking action on a small part of your dream—that you can do *right now*—that gives you some of the feeling of your dream.

For example: Let's say that your dream is to travel to France, to Provence. You cannot do that right now for whatever reason. So, a touchstone might be to watch a video about Provence. Or it could be cooking a French dish. Or finding some French lavender to smell. Or going to an art museum near you to look at Impressionist paintings.

Another example: You are curious about playing with erotic bondage. You are not sure how your partner feels about that. So, a touchstone might be to order some books, so you can learn more. You could get Kindle books since they are more private. Then you will have more information about the subject and also about how to approach your partner, when the time comes to have the conversation.

Touchstones are amazingly effective. Try them even if you feel that there is little hope. Do not fall into this pit: You can't have it all, so you pout and make sure that you have nothing. If you watch yourself and the people around you, you will see this all the time: Because they cannot have the whole enchilada, people make sure that they are completely miserable by insisting that they have nothing. Be ruthlessly honest with yourself here: Catch yourself if you are cutting off your nose despite your face.

- Review the resistance pitfall.
- Which touchstones can you create for yourself today?

## The fear pitfall:

Take the emotional risk of exploring more aspects of sex that interest you.

It is often scary to do that. Feel the fear and do it anyway. Here's a crazy and effective exercise:

Let your "future you" that is on your deathbed actually yell at your "present you" for not taking actions towards your dreams and goals. You do not actually have to yell out loud.

## Two useful questions about exploring:

- What is the worst that can happen if I do this?
- What is the best that can happen if I do this?

Then actually visualize the good outcome. Feel the good feelings inside yourself. Really focus on the details of your vision.

- Where are you?
- Who are you with?
- What scents do you notice?

- What are you doing?
- What are you feeling?

Those details will help you find the goals to strive for and the steps to take.

# Nonsexual Benefits of Cialis

## The Nonsexual Benefits of Daily Cialis

What are the nonsexual favorable effects of Cialis on the body?

How will Cialis help you enjoy better all-around well-being?

Why does an ED medication have benefits for general health?

### Case Study:

Peter is a busy plumber in his 50's. He has had lifelong issues with depressive moods. He tried antidepressants previously but did not like their impact on his sexuality and his weight. So, at this time, he was just putting up with his flat moods.

He also was unhappy about a decrease in his erections over the past few years. Sometimes they would be firm enough to start intercourse with his girlfriend but would fade soon after, never to return. Sometimes they were insufficient to have intercourse altogether.

He came to my office and was started on DC. He was enthusiastic from the start. He was surprised at the speed of the improvement of his sexual function. Later on, he noticed that he was more cheerful. His mood was more upbeat and positive. He told me: "I had forgotten how good it feels to feel good!"

## Did you know that Cialis improves your general health?

Cialis is a multi-faceted medication that has an astounding number of nonsexual health benefits. My patients are surprised when I tell them that Cialis is good for their all-around health, as well for their sex life.

When we think of Cialis, we automatically think of the sexual benefits. Sex is often considered to be a frivolous and nonessential part of life. So, the drug Cialis is often not taken seriously. It is not considered a "real" medication. Our puritanical society may say that any drug that enhances sex is a frivolous drug.

However, research continually finds more ways that Daily Cialis improves general health and also treats other health problems. It supports the body in staying younger and healthier. You will feel better in many aspects of your mind and body. These other health benefits apply to both women and men.

## Are you curious about research and statistics, like me?

It will amuse you that studies involving Cialis are tricky because you cannot completely make them double blind studies for the men. Men typically can tell when they are on Cialis by the sexual effects. So then, how do you test Cialis against placebo? It will be interesting to see how researchers manage that issue.

When you research these topics, you need to remember that Viagra and Cialis have the same mechanism of action. Much research is done on Viagra and will also apply to Cialis. Some research is done on Cialis only.

## How can Cialis accomplish all these very different things?

Think about it: Just like Cialis increases blood circulation in the penis, it increases it everywhere else too. So, the brain, the heart, the lungs, the muscles, the intestines, the skin, the kidneys, and everything else in the body receives more blood. And that is a good thing!

The body functions better with improved circulation. It heals better. It can withstand more stresses, such as the decreased oxygen at high altitudes.

With better blood flow, there is less inflammation in the body. And we all know how important that is! Inflammation causes many illnesses, health problems, and signs of aging.

## Is this information really proven?

All the astounding benefits below are from published scientific research studies. You can look them up on PubMed. Many topics are early studies. Some research used humans, some used rats and hamsters. More evidence will be needed to prove the definitive efficacy for each of the specific purposes. Do keep on the lookout for more of these astonishing research results.

# What all does Cialis achieve?

## For the heart:

- Better cardiovascular health, for the heart itself as well as the arteries.
- It helps to lower blood pressure.
- Research indicates that there is no increased risk of heart attacks.
- Men on Cialis do better after heart attacks.
- Reduces markers of cardiovascular disease.
- Helps with heart failure.
- Reduced myocardial infarct size in rats.
- It is considered "heart protective" in research studies

## For the lungs:

- Daily Cialis is a standard treatment for pulmonary arterial hypertension for women and men.
- May help with COPD.
- May help with asthma.
- Anecdotal reports of better, more restful sleep.
- Improves performance for athletes.
- Improves physical performance at high altitudes.
- Easier and quicker acclimatization to high altitudes; for us skiers, hikers, and climbers.
- Helps treat altitude sickness.

## For mental health:

- Significant antidepressant effect.

- Possibly in part due to increased blood flow to the brain.
- May increase dopaminergic activity in the brain.
- Helps with sexual problems due to SSRI antidepressant medications.
- May reduce anxiety.
- Improves libido, which in turn improves male moods.

## For the brain:

- Possible delay of onset and improvement with Alzheimer's.
- Helps with functional recovery after ischemic stroke.
- Possible neuro-protective treatment for ischemic injury to the brain.
- May help with memory.
- May help with jet lag although researched only in hamsters so far.

## For pain:

- Possible adjunct treatment for chronic pain.
- Part of a pain management plan, especially for nerve pain such as sciatica, and diabetic and other neuropathies.

## For the colon:

- In mice, Viagra reduced the number of polyps in the colon by 50%, which would result in fewer colon cancers.

## For mothers and babies:

- May help with preeclampsia, a serious complication of pregnancy.
- Helps with underweight babies in utero so they grow better.

## Overall benefits:

- Reduction of inflammation throughout the body.
- Daily Cialis is associated with lower cholesterol.
- It may help with Metabolic Syndrome.
- May help with weight loss by converting white fat into beige fat, which aids in burning fat.
- In view of the many varied effects of Daily Cialis, it may be an anti-aging medication.

## Cialis in recent research:

- Helps treat throat cancers by boosting the immune cells. Possibly colon cancer and other cancers too.
- Improves the symptoms of Multiple Sclerosis, Muscular Dystrophy, Raynaud's, and Parkinson's.
- Can help Restless Leg Syndrome, probably via increasing dopamine.
- Seems to help ED in spinal cord injury patients.
- May boost immune response to bacteria and viruses.
- Helped with liver transplants and liver cirrhosis.
- May help with colitis.
- Appears to help with kidney stones and kidney problems.
- Possible improvement of Chronic Prostatitis.

- Helps with sexual problems due to medications for high blood pressure.
- Helps with sexual problems due to medications for prostate enlargement.

## Some benefits are due to a better sex life:

- Research has shown: higher relationship satisfaction reported by *both* partners.
- The man's partner is happier in the relationship.
- The man's partner is more satisfied with the couple's shared sex life.
- Both partners feel younger.
- The couple enjoys the emotional benefits of the sexual activity.
- The female partner appreciates the increased connection that comes from sex.

# Antidepressant Action

Where do depressive moods affect your quality of life?

When do *you* feel less than positive and sparkly?

How can DC help your depressive moods?

## Case Study:

Roberto is a construction worker in his 50's who never had issues with his erections nor with his moods in his younger years. However, he had noticed that both had slowly been declining over the past few years.

His doctor and his friends told him that this is "normal for his age." However, in my medical practice I do not use that phrase. I want my male patients to be their optimal best at all ages!

We started him on DC and found his perfect dose. DC surprisingly can improve depressive moods in remarkable ways. Roberto did experience the happier moods. And of course, he was also happy that his sexual function was better.

During our visits we also talked about other ways for him to keep his sexuality and his moods improved. He feels that we used a holistic way to work on his issues, and he values that approach.

## Do *you* feel depressive moods?

- Feeling bleak or flat
- Not bubbly

- Not on top of your game
- Not feeling juicy
- Not feeling creative
- No joy in thinking about the future
- Not having fun
- Feeling low

## Challenge these myths:

- Men should man up and quit complaining.
- Men should put up and shut up.
- Sexual dysfunction is inevitable and happens to everyone.
- The world supports that unfortunate belief. Everyone around the man— spouse, friends, doctors—all spout that myth.

What are *your* beliefs about middle-aged men?

## How does DC work as an antidepressant?

- There are several mechanisms of action: Most likely it is a combination or a synergy of these different factors.
- Cialis appears to influence the dopaminergic pathways in the brain. Dopamine makes us happier.
- DC has a significant anti-inflammatory effect. It appears that inflammation is associated with depression.
- There is increased blood flow to the brain and within the brain.
- There is a small increase of testosterone which, in turn, promotes positive moods.

- DC promotes a strong libido which will improve depressive moods.
- Research indicates possible reductions in stress and anxiety with DC.
- Research has shown: Cialis and Viagra—across different cultures—improve confidence, relationship satisfaction, and self-esteem.

## How does DC improve depressive moods via better sexuality?

- When DC improves erections in a man—especially when there has been no or very little erectile function for some time—that will definitely cheer him up!
- With DC he often has more spontaneous erections again, either partial or full. It can definitely improve a man's outlook on life when his penis becomes more responsive.
- Men tend to be unhappy when their sex life is unhappy. They tend to feel good when their sex life is good. DC promotes good sexual function, and hence, a better sex life.
- DC provides increased sexual confidence.
- Research has shown: When a man takes DC, both partners report higher satisfaction with the relationship.
- It makes sense that a happier partner would make the man happier. And that a smoother relationship would make his life better.

## See a psychiatrist for major depression:

- If a man has a serious and severe clinical depression, then he needs to see a psychiatrist.

- This is called a major depression and needs to be treated seriously.
- If this is the case for you, do not self-medicate, and do get the proper care by an appropriate professional promptly.
- It may be essential for you to take antidepressant medication.

## Sexual side effects of antidepressant medications:

- Decreased libido or sexual desire
- ED, decreased sexual function
- Difficulty reaching orgasm
- Diminished orgasm
- Loss of sexual excitement
- Loss of sensation

## Help for the sexual side effects of antidepressant medications:

- DC significantly helps men with sexual function issues from antidepressant medication.
- There have been research studies on this topic.
- So, even in severe depressions, DC could likely be a useful addition to the antidepressant medications.

## Sexual desire and depressive moods:

## Low libido can be a cause of depression in men:

- One way that DC improves mood and decreases depression is by improving his libido.
- Men are different than women that way.
- When a man does not feel sexual desire, then he does not feel on top of the world.
- When he does not feel like a fully sexual man, then he does not feel masculine.
- When he is not sexually confident, then something is lacking in his life.
- When he does not take delight in attractive people around him, then he feels flat.

## Depression can cause low libido:

- This is the converse of low libido causing depression:
- When a man is depressed, his sexual desire is usually unsatisfying and, well, depressingly low.
- When his mood is off, then his sexual juiciness is also not present.

So, can you see how there is a positive or a negative feedback loop?

Which do you choose?

Which do you think makes for a better quality of life for the man?

Can you see why a doctor might want to consider DC therapy for a man with depressive moods? It is so satisfying to see men in my practice start to bubble and sparkle as their positive moods and vital libido come back. Men—and the ones who love them— don't know how easy it can be to make such a big difference.

## Here is what I say to you:

Do not go gentle into that good night! Fight, fight...for the buoyant life and for the sexual vigor that can be yours via DC.

# Athletic Performance

How could a sex pill help athletes?

Why would Cialis improve physical performance?

What is being studied about athletes and Cialis?

When you read about Viagra or Cialis being taken for athletic performance, you will notice that, so far, much of the research has been done on Viagra, not Cialis. However, both medications work via the same mechanism in the body so the research results are assumed to apply to both.

## How does Cialis work for athletes?

- It increases the effectiveness of a workout due to increased vasodilation which is mediated by nitric oxide. Therefore, circulation is increased, and more oxygen gets to the muscles, lungs, and other tissues.
- Improved blood flow to the lungs increases exercise capacity.
- It causes mild elevation of the testosterone level which is mostly due to the decrease of estrogen. Testosterone is less effective in the presence of estrogen.
- Higher testosterone leads to an increase in muscle mass and strength, and improved performance.

## Studies have shown:

- In runners who sprint: Cialis decreased the time to get to peak power.

- So, Cialis could be useful in sports where it matters how fast you get to maximum power output.
- C and V also activate muscle satellite cells which enable muscle repair and adaptation.

## In the future, athletes may use Viagra and Cialis for:

- Faster recuperation from a workout.
- Increased peak force.
- Increased nitric oxide, increased circulation.
- Increased endurance for older athletes.
- Increased endurance for recreational athletes.

Please note that this is an off-label use of Cialis and Viagra. That means that the FDA has not approved it for this purpose. So, you need to talk to your doctor before using it for this and any other off-label purpose.

Men sometimes worry that they will have random arousal and inappropriate erections if they take C in a nonsexual setting. However, since you still need the usual sexual stimulation to get hard, this actually does not happen.

More research is constantly being published. You can obtain more detailed, up to date information via search engines like Google and PubMed.

# Cialis at High Altitude

When have you felt not-quite-right, or even miserable, at high altitude?

How would you like to have better athletic performance when you are in the mountains?

What would you do with that benefit: Skiing, hiking, climbing, cycling?

## At high altitude, Cialis and Viagra do two things:

- Help people feel more normal who otherwise would suffer.
- Help athletes attain a better performance.

These benefits apply to women as well as men.

Research has shown that Viagra and Cialis improve athletic performance at high altitude. It is not yet a routine recommendation for women and men to take these medications when they go to high altitude. However, it may well become more common in the future as more research is done.

Some of the studies were done with Viagra. However, since Cialis and Viagra work the same way in the body, and since Cialis is so much more convenient due to its longer action, probably Cialis will be the most-used medication for this purpose.

In a study of bicyclists at high altitude reported in the *Journal of Applied Physiology*, some cyclists improved as much as 45% with Viagra. Some cyclists improved a great deal, while some did not improve much. It appears almost as if there are responders and non-responders. It will be fascinating to follow this research in the future.

Dr. Peter Hackett, famous high-altitude researcher, has investigated Cialis and Viagra in high mountains. In many climbers, the blood vessels in the lungs constrict at high altitudes. However, with Viagra and Cialis, they are wide open. He did a mini-study with four repeat climbers on Mount Everest. They all improved their times to summit. One climber cut his time from nine hours to less than four.

**Viagra and Cialis are even used in the emergency room in combination with other medications for problems of high altitude.** It is important to note: For actual high-altitude sickness you really need an experienced doctor or emergency room immediately. This is a really serious condition.

Don't use these medications for this purpose without getting cleared by your doctor because this is not yet an accepted use for them.

However, if you love the mountains and want to feel good even when first arriving there, talk to your doctor about taking Daily Cialis for a few days beforehand and while you are up there.

**And if you are an athlete who will be at altitude, talk to your doctor too.**

# Is Cialis an Anti-Aging Medication?

What is an anti-aging medication?

How would an anti-aging medication apply to you?

Where have you been skeptical about anti-aging miracles?

Which ways would you like your body to feel a little younger?

## What is an anti-aging medication?

All through history there has been a search for the Fountain of Youth or for a magic pill to turn back the clock of aging, with all its attendant complaints. Many medications and supplements and regimes are touted as the perfect anti-aging modality, except they usually do not actually work well.

With all the many and varied benefits of DC, it will be fascinating to see the future research. My own impression is that Cialis may well be seen as an effective anti-aging medication in the future. This does not mean that you take it and suddenly you are 25 years old again. It means that you feel better and are more functional because the Daily Cialis improves your physiology.

Scientifically, anti-aging means the process of preventing, slowing, or reversing physiological aging in the human body.

## About the scientific studies:

- Many of the above-mentioned effects of Cialis appear to apply to both women and men.
- Some of the scientific studies use Viagra, some use Cialis.

- The results of the studies should apply to both medications since their mechanism of action is the basically the same.
- Some of the studies were done on animals, and some on humans.

## The underlying principles:

- Just like it increases blood flow to the penis, Cialis increases circulation to the rest of the body for many benefits.
- Cialis reduces inflammation throughout the body.

## What can Cialis do?

Can Cialis help men and women keep their bodies healthier so that they can live longer, with fewer health problems and with a better quality of life?

I think so.

And you may agree as you read the following lists of current early research.

## Benefits for your cardiovascular system:

- Improves circulation by widening the arteries.
- Improves arteries and the endothelium of the arteries.
- Improves plaque in arteries.
- Improves microcirculation everywhere in the body, including the heart.
- Reduces inflammation everywhere in the body, including the arteries.

- Reduces markers of cardiovascular disease: Reduces C-Reactive Protein and Vascular Cell Adhesion Molecules.
- Improves recovery from strokes.
- Improves heart function, helps with preventing heart failure.
- Improves cardiovascular and exercise performance in some athletes. This could help many of us to exercise more effectively.
- Can help keep blood pressure lower.

## Mental and emotional benefits:

- Studies suggest that Viagra and Cialis can boost memory and learning skills.
- Can reduce pain.
- Has antidepressant action.
- Improves relationships.
- Men live longer when in relationship.

## Benefits for men:

- Can cause a small increase in testosterone.
- Can cause a decrease in estrogen in men. Estrogen is bad for men.
- Men and their partners have more sex.
- Sex is a huge contributor to good mental, emotional, and physical health.
- Improves prostate health.
- Improves BPH symptoms.
- Decreases urinary and bladder problems.

- Men get up fewer times at night to go to the bathroom.
- So, the men get better sleep, and their partners do too.

## Specific effects:

- In diabetics: Reduces inflammatory chemicals and improves fasting glucose levels.
- Less platelet aggregation on a cardiac stent.
- Has anti-tumor growth properties; used to treat some cancers.
- May boost immunity to viruses and bacteria.
- Converts undesirable white fat cells to the better beige fat cells which may help with abdominal fat and its health implications.
- May help with colitis.

## How can Cialis do so many different things?

This list is so long and so varied that Cialis can sound like a patent medicine that promises a cure for absolutely everything. However, when you think about how many health problems are due to inflammation and poor circulation, then this list makes sense.

## The story about inflammation:

Chronic inflammation is thought to lead to periodontitis (gum disease), atherosclerosis, hay fever, rheumatoid arthritis, and maybe even some cancers. Also, inflammatory bowel diseases, such as colitis and diverticulitis are connected with the inflammatory response; as are chronic prostatitis and interstitial cystitis. Inflammation is also linked to diabetes, gout, arthritis, and Alzheimer's.

Inflammation is closely connected with the progressive decline that we call aging. It is thought to be both cause and effect. Individual variation in inflammation is connected with environmental and lifestyle factors. If there is a way to decrease inflammation, then there will be a slowing of the degenerative aging process.

The term *inflammaging* has been used to refer to the chronic, low-grade inflammation that is connected with aging. Generally, age-related diseases have inflammatory causes. Older people with less inflammation live longer than those who have more.

More and more research is demonstrating the connection between inflammation and aging. There is more research in the works about how to reduce inflammation for better health.

Cialis and Viagra have been shown to reduce inflammation in general. Some research shows that they specifically may help to decrease the damaging effects of inflammation in human beings.

It is my belief that, with the benefits of both the anti-inflammatory action and the increased blood circulation, Cialis may well be considered a significant anti-aging drug in the near future.

## The story about blood circulation:

The same way that Cialis increases blood circulation to the penis, it also creates better circulation to every other part of the body. This increased perfusion is how it helps with various heart problems and how it shows promise for stroke treatment. There is some evidence that Viagra and Cialis, taken daily, may help prevent heart attacks and strokes.

Aging is associated with reduced blood circulation. Therefore, increased circulation can improve many of the symptoms of aging. Better blood flow throughout the body—the brain, the heart, the muscles, and the tiny peripheral blood vessels everywhere—will improve many markers of aging.

This improved micro-perfusion can decrease joint pain such as many experience with osteoarthritis. It can improve cognitive functioning of the brain. It can also give increased physical stamina for exercising more effectively.

## How does "feeling younger" make a difference?

DC already makes men feel younger by helping them have more and better sex. It makes their partners feel younger for the same reason. One of my patients said to me, "You've taken 20 years off my age." Feeling younger—by reducing stress levels—may actually help your body's physiology to act younger.

# Women and Cialis

## Sexual Cialis for Women?

How do Cialis and Viagra affect women for sex?

Why would a woman use them for sex?

What could the future uses be?

## Is Cialis useful for women?

The answer is: Yes and No.

## For sex:

For dramatic sexual benefits, unfortunately, the answer is No. However, there are some indications in the research that in certain conditions there can be some benefits. Hopefully there will be more studies and more information forthcoming in the future.

The fact is that Viagra and Cialis do *not* have the impressive sexual effect on women that they do on men. However, some studies suggest that in some situations women can derive some good.

## Women with low sexual desire:

For female sexual arousal disorder (FSAD): This issue tends to be multifactorial and complex. So it usually requires a variety of interventions in different ways.

FSAD involves both the body and the mind. In the body there can be problems with vaginal lubrication and engorgement of the vagina, vulva, and other sexual tissues. Mentally and emotionally there can be a variety of barriers to the desire for and enjoyment of sex.

Viagra and Cialis increase blood flow to the pelvis—and the rest of the body —in women just like in men. But women have less PDE5 – which causes Viagra and Cialis to work - in the vaginal and clitoral tissues than men have in the penis.

Studies suggest that: When the woman's sexual issue is more about actual physical and genital arousal problems, Daily Cialis has been proven to be helpful. This effect can apply to women who have type 1 diabetes. Presumably this same effect could be accomplished with Viagra as well, except it would last for a shorter period of time than Cialis.

If the problems are more about actually getting interested in sex and getting aroused, no clear benefit has been shown from Cialis or Viagra.

What if a woman just does not notice her feelings—both physical and emotional—of being turned on?

If women feel a general lack of attention to sexual cues, the combination of testosterone plus C or V can improve their genital response and their subjective sense of sexual function.

Initial research as well as anecdotal reports show: Some women do feel some flushing, glowing sensations and warmth in the pelvis. They also described a mild swelling of the clitoris and labia from the increased blood flow. These effects are ascribed to both Viagra and Cialis.

Anecdotal reports suggest that some women felt that they enjoyed sex more and reached orgasm more easily with Cialis. They felt that their sexual function was improved.

## Here is an interesting research study:

The Berman sisters, Dr. Jennifer, a urologist and Dr. Laura, a therapist, published a 12-week, double-blind, placebo-controlled study in 202 postmenopausal women with FSAD.

These women were given 50 mg of Viagra. The dosage could be adjusted from 25 to 100 mg.

They reported increased genital sensations with intercourse and/or foreplay. They also had increased satisfaction with intercourse and/or foreplay.

My interpretation: Interestingly the women either still had sufficient estrogen and testosterone or were on estrogen and testosterone therapy. The presence of sufficient hormones likely significantly enhances the effect of the Viagra.

## In summary:

- C and V do not appear to be miracle sexual drugs for women, like they are for men.
- However, they do help some women to some extent.

- In the future, we may find out more information about making it more effective for women's sexuality.
- Women tend to have the same side effects that men have.
- And the same risks apply to them.
- These prescriptions would be an off-label use of the medications.
- This means that they are not officially approved for these purposes.
- It is important that a woman work closely with her physician to assure safety and efficacy.

# Benefits for Wife or Girlfriend

How can my partner's DC make me happier?

Why is the Daily Cialis not just for him?

Why would a woman want her man to take Daily Cialis?

## Case Study:

Richard is a tall and good-looking man in his late 50's. He is a successful CPA and loves his hiking trips in the mountains. He and his wife Nancy are very involved in their church.

You would not have known from looking at him that he felt frustrated and less than a man due to his lack of erections. He felt badly about disappointing his wife. He was avoiding sexual situations with her.

She, in turn, was trying to be supportive of him but she missed sex and intercourse.

He had tried Viagra and that worked okay for his erections. But he hated the flushing, stuffy nose and blue vision. And Nancy really disliked having to plan ahead for sex by taking the pill and then waiting for it to take effect.

She felt inadequate, as if she were not sexy enough to get him aroused. And, every time he needed to take the pill, she was reminded of that. They were in a difficult relationship dynamic.

When Richard came to my office and was started on Daily Cialis, he felt so relieved and happy to be fully sexually functional again. He had some side effects with indigestion, and we worked on that problem.

Now he has a good libido and is sexually attracted to Nancy. He feels free to fully express that attraction, which she loves to receive. She feels sexy and desired.

On DC, his erections are reliable almost all the time. He can relax and enjoy sex again. He can please his wife now and bask in that glory. And for Nancy, sex is "natural" again. There is no waiting. They make love whenever they wish.

They are having their Best Sex Ever!

This story is not unusual. This scenario unfolds with frequency.

## Women can have the Best Sex Ever in midlife:

- Many women report that they are having the best sex of their lives in their 50's and 60's, and even later.
- The time around menopause can be a rich sexual life stage for women.

## What helps women have Best Sex Ever:

- *Creating* the sexual activities that they *really like.*
- Enjoying their own sparkling libido.
- Focusing on creating their own happiness in all of life.
- Feeling full of juicy life force.
- Exercising their bodies, in any way, to raise libido.
- Taking responsibility for their own happiness in everyday life.

- Taking bio-identical hormones if appropriate.
- Sexual thoughts and fantasies as well as actual sex create a positive feedback loop so that women feel more sexual desire.

## Key to women's turn-on:

A woman may have a flash of arousal that is:

- So tiny that she may not notice it unless she is looks for it.
- So fleeting that she may miss it.
- So brief that both partners need to move into an erotic space within just a couple of minutes.
- So subtle that she may not recognize it as arousal unless she looks for that.

## Women:

## When you feel that subtle and fleeting feeling of arousal:

- You need to tell him right away.
- You need to pounce on him right away.
- You need to start the sex that you want.

## Men:

## When she reports her turn-on:

- Drop what you are doing immediately.
- Start kissing and touching her.

- Realize that you may only have 3 minutes before her feeling fades.
- Realize that she is not playing a game to control you.
- Realize that this is just how women's desire can express itself.

When women have sexual desire, it is wonderful for their partner to meet them in that juicy love space. However, many men find that there has been some decline in their own sexual desire or sexual function or both. Then it is a great gift for the woman if the man is proactive to be on top of his game sexually.

## If her partner is on Daily Cialis, a woman appreciates these sexual benefits:

- She feels more comfortable initiating sex when she wants it.
- She feels more comfortable asking for intercourse.
- She has the pleasure of anticipating good sex.
- Both partners know that chances are good for the erection to work.
- She can have spontaneous sex.
- There is no need to wait for pill to work.
- For many women (and men) this feels like a more "natural" way for initiating sexual play.
- The quality of the sex is better.
- He is more sexually confident, which is a turn on for her.
- If she enjoys sexual intercourse, then she is more likely to get that with ease and predictability.
- Both enjoy the pleasure of their connection.

- Sex is good for both men and women's general health, as well as for their physical and emotional well-being. So more sex means better health for both.

## Women benefit from the man's better prostate health:

- He will have fewer of the prostate and bladder symptoms that make him—and her—feel older, such as him having to run to the bathroom frequently and urgently.
- She will sleep better because he is getting up fewer times at night to go to the bathroom.
- These beneficial prostate and bladder effects will be even more useful in the future because prostate problems get worse as men get older.

## Women benefit from their partner's Daily Cialis in nonsexual ways:

- He feels younger and acts younger.
- This is contagious: She feels younger too.
- Research has shown that both partners report greater happiness in their relationship.
- He may well live longer and be healthier due to DC's protective effects on the heart as well as other beneficial effects on general health.
- He has better moods.
- He fully feels his life force and life energy.
- He is a more fun and sexy partner.

# Women's Fears—and Hopes

How does the use of Cialis impact the wife or girlfriend?

What fears do men and women have about Viagra and Cialis?

Where can Cialis be used to improve the relationship?

## Case Study:

Gary is a 49-year-old man with unreliable erections and low sexual desire. He was feeling "less of a man" since he was not pursuing sex with his wife. He was also worried about his wife because she was not getting everything she wanted during sex. The problem was that his erections often faded during intercourse and would not come back.

The Daily Cialis therapy worked quite well for him. After only 5 days on Daily Cialis, he already felt his sexual function and sexual desire returning. This response is not unusual. "Doc, how can that happen so fast?" he asked me.

The fact is that Daily Cialis can begin to be felt very soon. Gary was so happy to feel like a real man again. He feels confidence as a man well as "cockfidence" as a good lover for his wife. She is grateful to him for taking action to make their marriage whole again.

## Women's feelings about Cialis and DC:

When men take Viagra or Cialis, it has complex effects on their partners and on the relationships. Many women want their husbands or boyfriends to take Cialis or Viagra. And the women are happy when the men do that, as in the case study above. The women love that they can have sexual intercourse again.

For some women, the as-needed Viagra or Cialis feels contrived or artificial. They do not like the idea of their boyfriend or husband taking a pill to get ready for sex. It feels unnatural to plan ahead or have to wait. Or they may just dislike the close association of the pill with their lovemaking.

Often these women strongly prefer Daily Cialis, rather than on-demand Cialis. Then the pill is not associated with intercourse. It's just another pill he takes every day. There is not the sense that they need a pill to make love. Sex can happen anytime. It feels more "like it used to feel" when they were younger. These gals are happy that the men can be ready anytime with Daily Cialis.

And when the men are not willing to take it, these women are unhappy because they really miss sex and intercourse.

## Couples talking about sex:

Cialis and Viagra can bring out the best in a man who is a giver and who makes a big effort to be a good lover. It can also bring out the worst if he is someone who takes and does not give. If the relationship is healthy, Cialis and Viagra can strengthen it further. If there are problems, the medications could make the problems more noticeable.

The woman may not know how to ask for what she wants; and the man may not know how to ask her. Some men of that generation—or of any generation—may not have gotten the message yet that the woman usually wants more than just the penetrative sex.

Couples can still have sex when the man has untreated ED. Some couples are content with that. And that is totally a reasonable option. They can use hands and mouths. However, there may not be sexual intercourse, and many men and women miss that. And he will not get hard from her caresses and oral sex on him, and many women miss that too. This is why both men and women may want the Daily Cialis or the Viagra on board.

## Women in middle age:

When a peri- or post-menopausal woman does not take estrogen as part of Hormone Replacement Therapy, it often is more difficult and uncomfortable for her to have intercourse. Also, typically she will have diminished sexual desire, or it can even be absent altogether.

She will also lubricate a lot less or not at all. Then if the couple does not use lube, she will be uncomfortable or have pain during intercourse. She may also feel vaginal irritation or pain afterwards. She may also get bladder infections or vaginal infections after sex which are almost always due to the lack of estrogen. These infections often can never be fully cured until she takes estrogen either vaginally or on her skin.

Additionally, there is the "use it or lose it" component. If she has not had anything inserted into her vagina for a while, it may take some time—plus lots of patience and lube—to build up that resilience again. A post-menopausal vagina can begin to constrict after even just two weeks of no penetration by anything.

Women may get comfortable and familiar with that no-intercourse kind of sex. Or with little or no sex. And it may feel alarming to them to consider the prospect of being sexual again. Therefore, even if a woman desires to have intercourse again, it may be a mixed bag for her; there may be emotional and physical discomfort in reviving that.

## Women may have fears about sex:

- Fear of not getting sex the way she wants it and needs it.
- Fear of "wham-bam-thank-you-ma'am" sex.
- Fear of not receiving enough nonsexual touch.
- Fear that there will only be sexual intercourse, and not the other play that she wants and needs.
- Fear that he will not take the time nor make the effort to really learn about her favorite sexual pleasures.
- Fear of not receiving enough oral sex.
- Fear of physical discomfort if he is not gentle and patient.
- Fear of physical discomfort if there is not enough lube and not enough estrogen.

## Women may have fears about the relationship:

- Fear of infidelity on the part of the man, if his sex drive and ability wake up again. Especially if she is not very interested in sex for whatever reason.
- Fear of infidelity on the part of the woman herself: If she wants sexual intercourse and he is not willing to take

Cialis to give her that, then she may feel a pull towards an affair.

- Fear of not feeling sexy enough or not feeling good enough: "If he needs a pill to get an erection, is it because I am not exciting to him?"
- Fear that the Cialis (or Viagra) will throw them out of synch sexually.
- Fear that he may again be capable of the pounding of intercourse while she is not.
- Fear that he may not get hard, even with Cialis on board. This could be because she does not realize that it is normal to still need stimulation by hands or mouth to have an erection.
- Fear that he will walk around with a constant erection because she does not realize that stimulation is still needed to get an erection.

## Fears that men may have:

- Fear that she does not understand how much a hard penis is a part of a man's identity. He is not being selfish or self-centered. It's just an important part of who he is in the world as a man.
- Fear that she may not understand that Cialis may increase libido. However, if his libido is really low, Cialis may not be enough to fix it, he may need testosterone, too. Either way she may feel confused and frustrated about his level of sexual desire.
- Fear that she may not understand that, even with Cialis on board, he still needs stimulation to get hard. His sexual functioning is just like it always was, he just responds better to the stimulation by hands or mouth.

- Fear that she may misunderstand his wish to take Cialis. She might not realize that he really does want to do this for her, too.

- Fear that she will not understand that his sexual desire is the same as his life force for him. If he does not feel sexually juicy, he does not feel alive. This can be very different than women's experience. And it can be very difficult for the women to truly understand.

- Fear that she may not believe that he really does find her attractive and sexy.

## Should the man decide, or should the couple decide?

When a couple discusses the issue of taking Viagra or Cialis, it helps grow the relationship intimacy. When both partners are involved in the decision, there is more of a team spirit.

A couple may not have the tools to easily discuss sexual needs and wants. You may find these topics to be tricky conversations. This situation is true for basically all couples of all ages. However, it is important to talk about these things as best you can. It helps if you always assume the *most positive interpretation* of what you hear from your partner.

Some men take Viagra or Cialis and keep it a secret from their partners. They may be worried that their partners might think less of them for needing that.

## If a man takes Viagra or Cialis secretly:

- When the woman finds out, she may worry that she was not sexy enough by herself.
- She may worry that he is taking it to have an affair.
- She may be sad that he has secrets from her.
- She may feel left out since she was not included in the planning for this medication.
- She may not understand why he wants the Viagra or Cialis. He may need to emphasize that he is doing that for her too.
- The man may feel inadequate for needing the Cialis and may hide it for that reason.
- There is also the risk of the pill getting the credit for some great lovemaking, rather than the people involved.

So you can see that the situation is more complex than just popping a pill. However, Cialis and Viagra are just tools: Use them for the best benefit for the both of you!

# Cialis for Women: Nonsexual Benefits

How different is Cialis for women than for men?

What is the research about Cialis and women?

Where could Cialis get used differently in the future?

## For the nonsexual benefits in overall health:

- Women receive comparable overall health benefits to those received by men.
- More studies have been done in men than in women since Cialis was, and is, mostly considered a medication for men.
- However, some studies have included women.
- It appears that the nonsexual effects are mostly analogous to the ones in men.

## For women as well as men:

There is one area where Daily Cialis is approved for women as well as men: For pulmonary arterial hypertension—PAH—which is high blood pressure in the lungs.

## The underlying principles for health benefits:

- They apply to both genders for general health:
- Improved blood circulation everywhere in the body.
- Reduced inflammation.
- Faster adjustment to high altitudes.
- Anti-aging benefits.

## Risks and side effects:

- Cialis has similar risks and side effects in both genders.
- If you are a woman and you want to take Cialis or DC for any reason, be sure to consult your doctor to make sure that this use will be safe and effective for you.
- Be sure to peruse the other applicable chapters in this book.

## What does Cialis achieve?

## For the heart:

- Better cardiovascular health, for the heart as well as the arteries.
- It helps to lower blood pressure.
- Research indicates that there is no increased risk of heart attacks.
- Men on Cialis do better after heart attacks.
- No analogous studies about heart attacks have been done on women yet.
- Reduces markers of cardiovascular disease.
- Helps with heart failure.
- Reduced myocardial infarct size in rats.
- Considered "heart protective" in research studies.

## For the lungs:

- Daily Cialis is a standard treatment for pulmonary arterial hypertension.
- May help with COPD.

- May help with asthma.
- Anecdotal reports of better, more restful sleep.
- Improves performance for athletes and weight lifters.
- Improves physical performance at high altitudes.
- Helps treat altitude sickness.
- Easier and quicker acclimatization to high altitudes— great news for us skiers, hikers, and climbers!

## For mental health:

- Significant antidepressant effect.
- Possibly due at least in part to increased blood flow to the brain.
- May increase dopaminergic activity in the brain.
- Helps with sexual problems due to SSRI antidepressant medications.
- Reduced anxiety in rats.

## For the brain:

- Possible delay of onset and improvement with Alzheimer's
- Helps with functional recovery after ischemic stroke
- May help with memory
- Possible neuroprotective treatment for ischemic injury to the brain
- May help with jet lag although researched only in hamsters so far

## For pain:

- Possible adjunct treatment for chronic pain
- Part of a pain management plan, especially for nerve pain such as sciatica, and diabetic and other forms of neuropathy

## For mothers and babies:

- May help with preeclampsia, a serious complication of pregnancy
- Helps with underweight babies in utero so they grow better

## Overall benefits:

- Reduction of inflammation throughout the body
- Daily Cialis is associated with lower cholesterol.
- It may help with Metabolic Syndrome.
- May help with weight loss by converting white fat into beige fat, which aids in burning fat.
- In view of the many varied effects of Daily Cialis, it may be an anti-aging medication.

## Cialis in recent research:

- Helps treat throat cancers by boosting the immune cells. Possibly helps treat colon cancer and other cancers too.
- Improves the symptoms of Multiple Sclerosis, Muscular Dystrophy, Raynaud's, and Parkinson's.
- Can help Restless Leg Syndrome, probably via increasing dopamine.

- May boost immune response to bacteria and viruses.
- Helped with liver transplants.
- Helped with liver cirrhosis.
- May help with colitis.
- Appears to help with kidney stones and kidney problems.

## Some nonsexual benefits are due to a better sex life:

- Better relationships!
- Research has shown: Higher relationship satisfaction is reported by *both* partners.
- The woman is happier in the relationship.
- The woman is more satisfied with the couple's shared sex life.
- Both partners feel younger.
- The couple has more sex.
- The couple enjoys the emotional benefits of the sexual activity.
- The female partner appreciates the emotional connection that comes from sex.
- The man has more masculine confidence.
- The partner also is pleased by the increased confidence.

## What's in the future for nonsexual use of Cialis for women?

Women's use of Cialis—both for sexual and nonsexual purposes —is a field where research will be fascinating. If this interest you, keep doing internet searches for new, cutting-edge scientific studies.

# Relationships and Affairs: Cialis and Couples

## Happier Relationships

Why would Daily Cialis fire up a relationship?

How could DC improve both partners' feelings about their marriage?

What does an erection pill have to do with a stronger marital bond?

## Case Study:

John and Karen are in their early 60's. They have been married for over 15 years. At the beginning of their relationship, both of them really enjoyed their fabulous sex life.

However, in the past few years they have started to bicker more. They get into fights more easily. Their love life is not so great because John's erectile function has been decreasing. Karen wants him to do something but doesn't know how to tell him that.

They start couple's therapy. Finally, with the therapist's help, Karen asks John to take action for the ED. It's hard for John to hear that but, he is also relieved that they are finally talking about the elephant in...the bed.

John comes to my office and starts Daily Cialis. He has a stuffy nose and headaches for the first couple of weeks. But he perseveres, and the side effects ease up. The main effects have been kicking in really well. His erectile function is perking up, and he is thrilled about that.

Karen is very grateful to him for taking the DC. And she is overjoyed that sex is so easy now. They appreciate each other as their sexual experience becomes more like it was at the beginning.

Their couple's therapy progresses so much more effectively now with the improved sex. They get along so much better with the good lovemaking.

There are still occasional erectile issues. But Karen and John have no problem working around that, since sex is basically just working so well.

Usually we think that only talking, and therapy, and "working on the relationship" can create more happiness for both partners.

## How could a simple pill make a difference?

## Research has shown that, when the man is on DC:

- Both partners report greater satisfaction with their relationship.
- Both partners report that finding independently from each other.
- Both partners report a higher sexual quality of life.

- This medication can have a positive effect for the man's wife or girlfriend.

## Researchers report that both partners are pleased that:

- Sex occurs more often.
- Sex can last longer.
- Sexual intercourse is easier.
- Both have more orgasms.
- It is easier for both to get to orgasm.

## You enjoy the subtler pleasures around sexuality:

- You both savor the anticipation of good sex.
- You appreciate the ease of initiating sex.
- You feel more carefree during lovemaking.
- You enjoy the pleasure of lovemaking and orgasms.
- You feel that the other one enjoys the sex more.
- And you are happy about that.
- Good sex makes you feel emotionally closer.
- You feel gratitude to each other for the sex and love.

## The man is happier:

- Daily Cialis has antidepressant effects.
- DC increases his Testosterone somewhat which has many positive benefits.
- DC has given him more sexual desire.
- Libido is the life force for men.

- DC has given him his life spark back via increased sexual desire.
- He has his masculine confidence back.

## The wife or girlfriend is happier:

- If she has been longing for having sex again or for more sex, she has a much greater chance of getting that now.
- If she has been doing the (possibly cautious) initiating of sex, she may enjoy that he is initiating more often too.
- A husband who is more sexually connected will be more affectionate in nonsexual ways too.
- A boyfriend who is not depressed will be more fun.
- He will have more energy for her and for their life.

## Your marriage benefits:

- His positive attitude creates a warm ambience in the marriage.
- He will have more patience and equanimity in his interactions with his spouse.
- He has more desire for intimacy and connection with his partner.
- He has more generosity of spirit for the family and the world.
- All these factors are major contributors to a loving relationship.
- Of course, other parts of the relationship also still need care and feeding; Cialis does not solve everything.
- However, with this stronger bond, you both will be more committed to nurture your relationship.

# The Danger of Affairs in Long-Term Relationships

How can you have Best Sex Ever in a long-term marriage?

Where can Daily Cialis help prevent infidelity?

What can improve sex for a middle-aged couple?

## Case Study:

Franco is a healthy man in his late 50's who was sent to my office by his wife, Laura. She was really unhappy about his constant irritability and bad moods. He also had trouble getting and sustaining an erection during sex, which probably contributed to his low moods. Laura was worried that she might be tempted to look for fun and sex outside the marriage.

Franco loves Laura and was willing to try Daily Cialis and testosterone both for his own sake and for hers. He was surprised when his moods improved by 80% in just a few days. And his erections and sexual confidence also improved quickly.

It was so satisfying to hear how their marriage had become sparkly again. They both definitely were in a positive feedback loop with good moods, good sex, lots of appreciation for each other, and more love. Laura was completely committed to their marriage again.

## What can you do about the danger of infidelity?

- The rates of marital affairs are at an all-time high.

- This applies to both women and men.
- Cialis and Viagra have been accused of contributing to marital affairs.
- Wives and girlfriends worry that the guy will use his reawakened sexual function elsewhere.
- They especially worry if they themselves are not interested in sex any more.
- This scenario does happen.
- But it also constantly happens that their guy just wants to connect more with them and make them happy.
- So, Cialis and Viagra also make relationships more fun and more connected.
- The boyfriend and the girlfriend, the husband and wife: Both have the power to use Cialis for greater bonding and more pleasure in the relationship.
- Both partners can take the initiative to create a stronger relationship.
- And Cialis as well as Daily Cialis are powerful tools for that purpose.
- Research has shown that when a middle-aged man takes DC, both partners are happier.
- A torrid affair makes for exciting drama, and some people are drawn to drama.
- However, a fulfilling long-term marriage really will make your life better in the long run.
- So, investing in that relationship really means investing in your present and future happiness.

## What about sexual excitement in a long-term relationship?

Eventually you lose the sexual excitement of the new relationship. You have that issue that Esther Perel talks about in her book *Mating in Captivity*:

- For sex to be exciting there has to be newness.
- However, when a couple has been together for a long time, then there is comfort and familiarity.
- These things feel nice but do not contribute to sexual heat

We get quite 'efficient' in getting each other off. We get into sexual habits and routines which work fine but are no longer exciting. We don't experiment with new and wild sexual toys or activities.

In a way, we have more to lose now. If we suggest something new, we risk that our partner makes fun of us. So we are hesitant to go outside the box. But then we also lose sexual excitement.

## Long-term relationships plus issues of middle age:

- People tend to gain weight.
- They may have less physically mobility.
- They have more aches and pains.
- Both partners may have less sexual desire.
- Both partners may have more depressive moods.
- The women have problems with vaginal lubrication, though that is easily fixed by using lube.
- Many men will start to have erection issues.

- These ED issues are depressing and discouraging so men find it difficult to take action for that problem.

## Sex in long-term relationships is improved with Daily Cialis:

### For you, the woman:

- Your partner is ready for sex anytime. So you can tune into your own spontaneous desires. Sex becomes more exciting again.
- There is no pill to take that requires waiting, like with Viagra.
- When he is ready for sex anytime, you avoid that contrived feeling.
- His sexual desire is better. It lifts a woman's spirits when she feels wanted. You both feel the excitement of attraction.
- You feel younger when he feels younger and more virile.
- DC has antidepressant properties via three different mechanisms. When he feels more cheerful, then you also feel happier.
- If you tackle your low libido, then your own life will be so much happier. Reading the happiness books and self-help books is okay. However, what really makes the biggest difference is feeling your womanly sensuality and your sexual satisfaction.
- It's time to take a break from all your resentments against him and against life.
- It's time to be an adult and create your sexual life the way you want, and to live life fully before you die.

## For you, the man:

- Your sexual performance is better. You regain your sexual confidence. You enjoy feeling your masculine self.
- That makes you feel younger. When you feel younger, she feels younger. And your relationship feels younger.
- When you have more sexual confidence, you are more fun to be with and you have more fun. You are more adventurous for creating sexual scenarios for the both of you.
- DC improves your libido, although testosterone does that even better. When you have more libido, and you have the maturity and wisdom to channel that libido to your partner, then you both are happier.
- You have fewer of those depressing prostate and urination issues. You feel younger that way too.
- If you make a big effort to figure out what works for her, then you will both benefit.
- And what actually works for her may be different than what you are believe you know! Put your ego on the back burner and just be curious.

## For you, the couple:

- As you have more sex, you feel more connected. And the more connected you both feel, the more sexual you are with each other. You start a positive feedback loop.
- You will squabble less and enjoy each other more when you have had sex recently.
- Working on the relationship goes better after sex. Make love before you talk.

- By being ready for sex anytime, you both feel younger: Back to the days when your bodies were always ready for sex, and there were no kids to get in the way. You can be playful again.

- When you have more juice with yourselves and with each other, you become more willing to share erotic fantasies and try to have them come true.

- You are both old enough and smart enough to realize that you will die someday—life is not forever—so you'd better live now. And it is now or never for those sexual fantasies.

- You have been together long enough that you know how to communicate. So you can talk about what works for you sexually and what does not.

- And: If it is difficult to talk, then it is time to learn— maybe with a sex therapist, or with books and videos such as those by John Gottman or Alison Armstrong.

- You are both realistic adults now: You realize that good sex is definitely a use-it-or-lose-it situation. So you make sex happen on a regular basis even if one or both of you is not exactly raring to go. You do it anyway because it is good for both of you and for your relationship.

- Both partners are more willing to do what's needed. So the man is more willing to take Daily Cialis for the sake of the marriage.

# Cheaper Than Divorce—More Fun Too

How can you two enjoy each other more?

How can a pill like Cialis save your marriage?

What can you two do to have more fun together?

## Case Study:

Back when I was still treating women before specializing in men:

Naomi was in her 50's when she came to me because she could not stand how badly she treated her husband. She noticed that she was constantly irritated at him and criticizing him. She was sure that he would leave her if she didn't shape up.

I realized that she was probably unhappy too because she was probably treating herself that badly too. And she felt so frustrated with herself for being unable to "shape up."

She was started on estrogen and progesterone. She could not believe how differently she felt. The sun had come out from behind the clouds. Life felt manageable to her now. She liked herself. She liked her husband and expressed that to him.

She said to me: "You saved my marriage!"

The best part for me: Her marriage was not saved by her needing to shape up or push herself to become someone else. Her marriage was saved because she was able to become her authentic healthy self again.

When men feel better about themselves while taking Daily Cialis, similar positive dynamics are at work.

## Is your mind or your body in control?

- Relationships are all about feelings and emotions.

- What controls those feelings and emotions?

- My experience in my office and in social conversations demonstrates that we underestimate the importance of biochemistry on our emotional life.

- We tend to think that emotions are all in the mind, and that we "should" be able to control them with our minds.

- However, the emotions are hugely controlled by hormones and neurotransmitters, which are biochemical messengers.

- In my practice I so frequently see dramatic shifts in patients' state of emotions with medications such as Daily Cialis or testosterone.

- These observations imply that our emotions are influenced as strongly—or more strongly—by biochemical changes as by emotional or spiritual work.

- I find this observation very humbling since we believe so strongly in the power of the mind.

- But what if the mind is really mostly influenced by the biochemical substances in the body?

- So, maybe a pill really could create change in a relationship!

## How can Daily Cialis save your marriage?

- More than one couple has told me that their marriage was saved by the information and prescriptions from their medical visits with me.

- I am a regular Medical Doctor with a strong psychological bent. I am not a therapist.

- However, in my medical practice both the body and the mind are addressed.
- Sexual issues in a marriage involve both the emotions and the body.
- The tricky part is that the biochemistry of the body strongly influences the emotions.
- Research has shown that both partners report higher satisfaction with their relationship when the man is on Daily Cialis.
- When the couple has fun in bed, then the rest of life also goes more smoothly.
- Good sex helps improve other facets of the relationship, such as the little and big stresses of everyday life.

## When I am talking to my male patients, there is always

- Awareness of their all-around well-being, as well as their sexual vitality.
- Awareness of this man as part of a couple.
- Awareness of supporting the happiness of the couple.
- You will notice this emphasis in this chapter and in this entire book.

## Solving andropause and menopause:

- It makes sense that andropause and menopause are a dangerous combo.
- Andropause is the man's life stage when his hormones start to decline, and he is no longer on top of his game.

- Symptoms of andropause include irritability and depressive moods, which are not good for relationships.
- Andropause also is a time of declining sexual desire and sexual function, which also causes stress for the man and for the couple.
- Menopause is when many women become less happy with themselves, their marriage, and the world.
- Back when I had female patients in my practice, it amazed me how often female hormone replacement would save marriages.
- With men, there is also a striking difference when men are on Daily Cialis and/or testosterone: Their moods are so much more positive and confident.
- When the man is on Daily Cialis, the woman can enjoy his higher level of *desire for her*.
- When andropause and menopause are appropriately managed with prescriptions by an experienced practitioner, then the couple really can have their best marriage ever and the Best Sex Ever.

## Women's challenge in menopause:

- Women's moods typically plummet in midlife.
- This impacts their own happiness as well the happiness of the people around them.
- It is a sad and vicious cycle when the woman cannot find ways to enjoy life.
- Then it is so easy to blame her husband.
- She may assume that the marriage is the problem, especially if it is a long-term marriage.

- However, leaving him is not necessarily the best thing for her own long-term happiness.
- Often, when the woman starts taking estrogen, the marriage suddenly feels better for everyone, including herself.
- Female hormone replacement therapy (HRT) does not solve everything, but it helps a lot.
- It is safer than commonly assumed.
- More than once, a patient has reported to me that her HRT saved her marriage.
- This can be because she is no longer so irritable to her husband, so he is happier.
- It can also be that on HRT she has a more positive outlook on life, including her husband. So she is happier with him again.
- HRT also helps if she has low sexual desire.

## Why a good marriage matters:

- Studies have shown that most of our happiness comes from the connections with the people around us.
- And of that, most of our happiness comes from our primary relationship.
- How things are going with our partner makes the biggest difference for our happiness in life.
- So it is very much worth your while to continually make it your focus to cherish your partner.
- And to keep finding more ways to nourish her and the relationship.

## One great tool for you—The Love Languages:

- Have you heard of the *5 Love Languages*®?
- Make sure you know what your partner's love language is.
- I will bet you that it probably is not what you think it is.
- If you want to be effective in having your partner feel loved, and if you don't want to waste your work on ineffective things, you have to actually figure out her love language with her.
- Once you know her love language, then you can figure out which actions will have the most impact for her.
- And then you'd be smart to do those things, even though they make no sense to you because your love language probably is different.

## Use the Love Languages together:

- The problem for women is that they focus too much on trying to guess how to make their partner happy, instead of making themselves happy.
- Your wife or girlfriend spends a lot of time and energy thinking about that.
- And also, she is always wondering how to "improve the relationship."
- If you work on that also—by yourself as well as jointly with her—you will gain many, many brownie points with her as well as a happier wife, happier relationship, and happier life.
- One easy and very effective way to do that is to get the book by Dr. Gary Chapman or go to the website about The 5 Love Languages.

## Other resources:

- Alison Armstrong's audio, YouTube videos, and live courses.
- John Gottman's books and YouTube videos.
- Esther Perel's work, especially her book *Mating in Captivity*
- If want counseling, you might consider choosing a therapist via the AASECT website.

## An exercise—How to enjoy yourself and your marriage again:

- Think about all the people you know who got divorced. What did they do once they were single again?
- Think about: What things would *you* do if you were single again?
- Typically, the list includes personal improvement and fun:
  - Going to the gym, getting slim and fit.
  - Dressing better, sharper clothes. Getting a nicer haircut.
  - Taking up a new hobby.
  - Getting out more. Being more social.
  - Doing more things with friends.
  - Sprucing up your home.
  - Traveling more.

## Here is your challenge:

- How many of those things on your list can you do now, even though you are married and plan to stay married?
- If you find yourself saying, "My spouse would never let me," think again.
- Could it be that you are using your spouse as an excuse for not stepping wholeheartedly into creating your own full life?
- Often spouses are more willing than we think.
- Sometimes it can be worth making a change in your life that means a lot to you, even though your partner is a little uncomfortable. Better to do that than get divorced. The partner usually adjusts.
- It can be scary to change things in your life but maybe that is what is needed.
- You could try changing some things about *yourself* and about *your* life to make yourself happier. Then see if that makes you happier in your marriage.

## This is your reward:

If you combine optimal biochemical well-being with emotional learning for each of you, then you both will reap synergistic results for greater happiness as individuals and as a couple.

The greatest rewards come to those who dare!

# Couples: How to Enjoy Daily Cialis

What is the best way to make the decision to start Daily Cialis?

Why does Cialis complicate some things in a relationship?

How do men and women see this medication differently?

## Case Study:

James is a quiet guy who works hard at his engineering job for the city. He is in his mid-fifties, has greying hair, and a bit of a pot belly. He was divorced, remarried a few years ago, and loves his wife Cheryl a lot.

Cheryl is a vivacious, curvy woman who is likes her work at the library. She enjoys sex and sensuality.

Both have noticed that they have been having sex and intercourse less frequently in the past year or two. His erections often are less firm, and sometimes fade during intercourse.

She is worried that he is not turned on by her any more. He is worried that she will look elsewhere for sex. He did not expect to have sexual issues until much later in life, so he is discouraged.

Luckily, they are both comfortable talking about relationship stuff, including sex. Over the course of a few weeks they gradually share their worries and concerns. They also do research online together and separately about ED.

Finally, they both decide that they are ready for him to try ED pills. He goes to his doctor and gets started with Daily Cialis. After a couple of adjustments in dosage, his erections are back to normal. They are both thrilled with their renewed sex life. And also, they are pleased that they worked through this issue as a team.

## Erection medications can be complex in a relationship:

- Often the prescription is written without discussion about the possible impacts on the feelings of the man and the woman.
- Sometimes the couple can get broadsided by their reactions to this new and unfamiliar dynamic in the relationship.
- Adding an erection medication to an ED situation can be straight forward—or not.

Sometimes a man gets a Viagra or Cialis prescription from his doctor, and he starts using it without any discussion with his wife or girlfriend. This situation can change the relationship dynamics and cause confusion.

Sex therapists say that one should not take ED medications to cover up distress or anger in the relationship. This approach certainly makes sense. However, it is also true that good sex can make the couple feel more connected so that relationship problems are easier to manage.

So it can be really great for the couple to talk about this issue of taking Viagra and Cialis. It can be really useful if both partners are involved in the decision to experiment with these medications.

Possibly they may want to have this discussion in the office of a sex therapist to get the best possible support.

It is useful to emphasize the experimental nature of this new medication when you talk. Both partners are learning about this new situation. Both partners can suggest different things to try, about the prescription and about the sex they are having with it.

## The reactions of men and women:

Many women are grateful to their partners for taking Viagra or Cialis. Now that the kids are grown and gone, the women are ready to focus on having fun with their man. They appreciate his willingness to do whatever it takes for their sex life to be as spectacular and special as possible.

There are plenty of women who would love for their partners to take those medications; however, for whatever reason, the men do not want to do that. Again, these situations can be very complex and might benefit from some sessions with a good sex therapist.

Sometimes men prefer to have their partner not know that they are taking the ED pills. They may worry that the woman will think less of them for needing a "crutch." The men may feel pressure to satisfy their wife or girlfriend with good sexual performance. However, they may be afraid of her reaction if she finds out about the V or C.

Sometimes women have negative feelings when their male partner is taking erection drugs. They may worry that they are not good enough or not sexy enough. Or they may feel that the relationship is not exciting enough for the man.

This is a tricky situation because often the man is taking the medication to provide the sex that he thinks she wants. Many midlife men have a reduced capacity to get hard when they want to. It does not mean that they are less attracted to their partner or that the partner is not sexy enough. So it is a good thing when a woman can appreciate a man for taking these medications—for both their sakes.

Some couples have settled into a stable "no sex" relationship. Or they may have very limited sex. Then, when he starts the erection meds and wants to have sex again, it can be confusing and uncomfortable for the woman. She may worry that he is involved with someone else. Or she may not want to have sex for various reasons, and now she feels pressured. She may also be curious about having sex again but may worry that she is too old for the hanky panky.

## To start having sex again:

Women—and men—may want to have better sex than they were having in the past. It is a big accomplishment in the relationship if both partners can suggest things to try, and the other partner is receptive and not defensive. While you both are newly experimenting with the C, you may be more willing to try other new things too. This may be a good time to dust off old fantasies and wishes. It may also be a good time to share your current fantasies and wishes.

## Never laugh when your partner shares intimate sexual secrets:

- When you both give each other loving permission to talk about anything, then the fun really starts big time for both of you!
- You are never obligated to do something, just because you talked about it.
- If something does not interest you, just say, "I'm not really into that right now."
- Do not say derogatory things about your partner's interests.
- Do not let them do that about yours.
- There are times when loving partners do things for each other that are not their favorite things.
- When you do that, it's like serving their favorite dinner even though it is not your favorite dish.
- Doing something just for them is a generous gift that you give when you feel ready.

## A good way to phrase a sexual request is:

"I love making love with you, and there is this thing that I'm curious about and might want us to try." It is helpful to emphasize that you are trying something, that you are experimenting. Neither partner is committing to this new thing— it is just an experiment. Nothing is wrong; things are good; you just want them to be even better.

## If you are thinking about using a sex therapist:

Remember the definition of a sex therapist: A therapist who can talk about everything, including sex. A good sex therapist will help the couple work on all sorts of issues, emotional as well as sexual. They definitely feel comfortable talking about sex, which is not true for every therapist. They have additional knowledge and training about sexual issues. A good way to find a sex therapist is via the AASECT website: American Association of Sexuality Educators, Counselors and Therapists.

# What If One Partner Has Low Desire?

How have you experienced discrepant sexual desire?

What can you do to create sensuality that works for both of you?

When have you enjoyed sex even though you did not expect to when you started?

## Can you have the Best Sex Ever in middle age?

Yes, it is true—you can! And it is not rare nor difficult—it is very possible. It does take focus and willingness to take action. One issue that can come up is that one of the partners has lower sexual desire than the other one.

## Discrepant sexual desire:

Couples of any age can have discrepant sexual desire, which means that one partner wants more sex than the other one. However, in midlife that situation becomes more frequent and more pronounced.

We tend to assume that it is the women who have low desire, and not the men. However, that is not always true. Men of any age can have also issues with low sexual desire. It can be associated with depressive moods. When men become middle-aged, they can have symptoms of andropause: Their testosterone drops, and the sexual desire and function declines.

Statistically, in our society, both men and women can be high-desire as well as low-desire partners. However, in my experience of midlife couples, low desire is more common in women. This could be due to the fact that the men in my practice are being treated to be in optimal health, so they have good libido.

Some women never have high sexual desire at any point in their lives. Sometimes their libido decreases with babies and children. When women start toward menopause, which can be as early as age 40 or before, their sexual desire can plummet. As they go all the way through menopause, their interest in sex can really diminish. Once you add the problems of dryness and lack of lubrication, plus other vaginal and bladder symptoms, sex can become very unappealing to them. All these issues are worse if the woman does not take hormones.

Long-term marriages are a separate but related situation: Many midlife people are also in long-term relationships. So then you have the two overlapping sets of problems: Midlife hormonal decline plus some ennui with the too-familiar partner.

Then add the increased illnesses and disabilities plus the increase in weight that may accompany middle age, and you have a perfect recipe for a sexual desert. Sexless marriages are a difficult and serious problem.

But it does not have to be like that! For plenty of women, sex becomes truly great with menopause. They feel liberated in many ways: No more child-rearing, less worry about what others think, a sense of now or never. Then, if you add Hormone Replacement Therapy plus information about vaginal lubrication products and sexual variety, they can really bubble with sexual juiciness and adventure.

## What can the couple do to optimize the sex life for both of them if the woman has low desire?

### What can the man do?

- Take out the trash! Really! Find out—don't assume that you know—which tasks she values most, then do them reliably. That way she may feel less stressed about her long To Do list.
- Don't push hard for sex. This is really hard to do. However, if she feels that she is being pressured, she will be so busy resisting that she won't even have a chance to feel her own occasional desire.
- Be a Sherlock Holmes and figure out what she likes in sensual pleasures. She may not know herself. So, ask her but also observe her. Which scenes in movies does she like? What comments of hers give you a hint?
- Look up the Five Love Languages and figure out which is hers.
- Talk with her and listen to her. Maybe you can even create some light-hearted conversation about something fun and sexy.
- Don't always push for your orgasm. Find ways to enjoy sensuality only— without intercourse—if that is what she wants.

## Be Good, Giving, and Game:

Make sure that you are being Good, Giving, and Game—as *Savage Love* recommends:

- Be good at your sexual skills and keep learning more.
- Be generous with giving oral sex, caresses, kisses all over.
- Be game: Be available to her when she wants sex even if it is inconvenient. Be willing to try things that she may like. Never say anything that could in any way be interpreted as negative.
- Always be positive and enthusiastic about anything coming from her as regards sex or sensuality.
- Never ever make fun of any of her fantasies or her desires.
- Always be positive about her body and how it looks and feels. Encourage her feel the nice sensations, rather than worry about how she looks.
- Make sure that your breath is fresh, and your body is freshly showered, with a really well washed, clean smelling butt.
- Consider taking Daily Cialis so that you are ready whenever she is.
- If you go into couples' therapy, go to a Sex Therapist. You can find them on the AASECT website. The reason for that: A sex therapist is comfortable talking about sex—as well as other topics—whereas many other therapists are not comfortable talking about sex. And they may not tell you that because they may not be aware of it themselves.
- Encourage her to make her lists for Date Night. Never make fun of any item on the list in the least little bit. This

is her learning about how to get into a sensual space. Women are different than men!

## What can the woman do if she has low desire?

### For your sex date:

- Go for what *you* want to experience with him. It's okay if he is not wildly enthusiastic—he'll live. For example: He has come and feels done with sex. But you want more. So position yourself so that he can give you oral sex for another half hour or hour.

- This is really important: Focus on feeling the sensations inside your body. Do not focus on how you look. Enjoy yourself. He is fine, no need to worry about him. Just focus on the yummy feelings.

- Does it help you to have a glass of wine—no more than that—or other things to relax? Then do use that, in moderation.

- This is also really important: Do you tend to say after sex: "That was great! We should do that more often."? That means that your brain does the common thing of not remembering pleasure. So you need to just get started with some sensual pleasure because the memory is not there to push you. Permit him to help you remember how much fun you had last time, and the details of what you enjoyed.

## For herself in daily life:

- Avoid popular media and women's magazines, which are basically always sex-negative, even if that is not immediately apparent. They encourage women to be sexy, rather than sexual. That is a subtle and significant distinction.
- Spend time with women friends who enjoy sex.
- Women sometimes worry about the scent of their genitals. Women's genitals have scent. So get over it and relax. Use plain water, often. Bidets (including the inexpensive toilet attachments from the hardware store) or "smart toilets" are great. Never use soap nor scented products on the vulva or vagina.
- Spend time and energy to have fun in daily life! Get Barbara Sher's *Live the Life You Love*. Read "Lesson 6: Resistance," first.
- Use that "Resistance" lesson also to get yourself more sensual fun.
- Move your body and get exercise in ways that you really like.

## For her well-being with hormones:

- Spend time with women friends who are on hormones: Estrogen / progesterone and testosterone.
- Educate yourself about and consider Hormone Replacement Therapy, including the small female amounts of testosterone.
- Find a doctor who is familiar with HRT and consult with them.

- Do not randomly google the topic of Hormone Replacement Therapy. You will get alarmist and worthless information. Choose your sources carefully. For example: Read the book "Estrogen Matters" by Dr. Avrum Bluming and Carol Travis PhD. Read the article on Hormonophobia by Dr. Abraham Morgentaler on PubMed. They question and disprove the study that scared women off hormones.

## What can you both do? Sensual Date Night!

You can start the habit of a sensual date night:

It works best to discuss this topic when you are both feeling happy and connected.

You will be talking about:

- This is different than the date night for dinner out or Netflix.
- This is specifically for connecting your bodies and erotic energies, as well as your hearts.
- How often you will have this. Once a week? More or less often?
- How much time? How long for the sensuality and sexuality?
- Maybe one hour? Maybe more or less?
- Then you put it into both your calendars.

## Be adults about Date Night:

You will both be adults about this:

- This means that you will not cancel for anything other than an emergency room visit.
- You realize that you will have resistance and you will do it anyway:
    o Because it is good for you.
    o And because it is normal to have resistance.
- You will also be adults in this way: You realize that it is wonderful to schedule a date.
- However, you can still have spontaneous sex play at any other time.
- And also, you are scheduling this event even though the scheduling process may feel new and a little uncomfortable.
- You will also act like adults in taking responsibility for creating activities that you enjoy.
- Especially for the low desire partner: Do think of things that you want to try or want to experience. No matter how silly or crazy, or how long or short.

## For the Low Desire Partner to create Date Night:

- Get a little journal or take notes on your phone about what works for you. You will not remember these details, so you need to write them down. Have the journal and pen handy during your date night so that you can write notes in the moment.
- Choose a realistic length of time for you. Better to have it be shorter and be really engaged, rather than longer and dreading it.
- Wear lingerie that *you* like. That feels good on *you*.

- Make a list in your journal—and keep adding to it—of what you need at the date night: Temperature of room, music, doors locked, etc.
- Make a list—and keep adding to it—of what you want from him for date night. Nothing is too trivial: You have to honor your irrational desires because sensuality is irrational.
- You may add things like: To shave, to shower and thoroughly wash his butt, brush teeth, to not drink much alcohol or similar substance, to rub your feet for 10 minutes, etc.
- These lists (or the combined list) may be a long list, and that is totally fine. Print it out so that it is visible to both of you.
- Make the list matter-of-fact and positive.

So very many couples have discrepant desire that it is really worth working on: This learning is your ticket to more fun and satisfaction together for the rest of your lives. So you might as well dive into it now!

# Spontaneous Sex Again!

How would you like to have sex anytime at all?

What do you need to have spontaneous sex?

When have you enjoyed having sex with no planning needed?

## Case study:

Shawn is a vital man in his 60's. He owns and runs a big farm. He has buddies that he hangs out with over beers at the sports bar. However, he and his friends do not talk about their sex problems.

He had some ED issues that were solved well by his use of Viagra. His girlfriend Lori was unhappy because it felt "unnatural" to her to need to take a pill for sex. She felt older and less attractive because her lover needed to take a pill to have an erection with her. She knew that this was not actually true, but the feeling remained.

So Shawn was happy when Lori found information from me about Daily Cialis. He got his prescription and was happy to start using it. Now he just takes the tablet every morning, with his other pills.

Now she is happy because their sex appeared to be unrelated to any pill. And Shawn also loves that, with the Daily Cialis, his sexual function is similar than when he was years younger. He feels that he is his normal and virile self again.

Do you dream of passion like in the movies, like in your youth? You see each other, you kiss, you breathe each other's scent. And then you cannot resist pouncing on each other for hot sex that leaves you breathless. You are ready for sex anytime and all the time. You get turned on at random times and you want sex then.

## You can have that spontaneous passion again!
Some people believe that sex should always be spontaneous. They do not like to plan ahead for sex. They feel that sexual feelings and activities should arise out of the desire in the moment. Those people may feel that taking Cialis or Viagra before the sexual activity feels contrived and artificial.

Impromptu sex is wonderful and fun and exciting. However planned sex dates are also very important. Both ways are good!

## What does spontaneous sex give you?
- You feel unfettered and free spirited.
- You feel young and sexy.
- You can flow with the energy of the moment and can enjoy sudden bubbles of erotic turn on.
- When you see a sexy picture and react with a buzz, you can follow that desire and have sex right then.
- After all the kids have left home, you are really appreciating this new freedom to make love anytime of the day or night.
- And also, you can really enjoy the freedom of making love anywhere in the house—wherever the mood strikes you.
- It gives you the freedom or permission to have a quickie.

- And: A quickie may give you the freedom or permission to do sex differently than your usual routine.

## How to have spontaneous sex with your partner:

- Couples that are dedicated to their erotic connection will negotiate ways to follow their sexy impulses, even when one partner is more in the mood than the other.

- Some couples have an agreement that, when one partner initiates, the other partner will go along with that, to whatever extent they choose.

- This is a tantric practice: You start making love anywhere in the spectrum of erotic activities, and end it anywhere. You don't always follow the usual pattern of foreplay, intercourse, orgasm, end.

- You can have quickies. The man may choose not to ejaculate every time. Instead he may do the tantric thing of channeling the sexual turn-on energy into something else: writing that chapter, going for a run, running that meeting. The woman can also choose to use her energy from the sexual play in similar ways.

- Look for more information about quickies in the chapter on that topic.

- These attitudes and practices give you the freedom to have a lot more sex—and a lot more creative, fun, irreverent sex.

- It probably did not escape you that Daily Cialis is the ticket to the option of spontaneous sex!

## How does Daily Cialis give you impromptu sex?

- When a man takes DC, he takes the pill on a regular schedule every day.
- He takes the pill whether or not sexual activity is planned for that day.
- Therefore, taking the pill and having sex play are completely unconnected and separate.
- For many men, this feels really good and really natural.
- Men feel sexually similar to their younger years. There is *not* that constant reminder of ED like when you have to pop a pill before sex.

## Women also love the unconstrained timing of lovemaking!

- When the man takes Daily Cialis, he is ready for her all the time.
- He does not need to rush off to find the little blue pill, and then they have to win for it to work.
- Many women feel more desired and desirable when the man is turned on by them more of the time—with an erection to prove it.
- If it feels artificial to you when he has to take the pill, then DC will feel more natural to you.
- Women have the opportunity to start to feel their tiny sparks of desire. Often erotic feelings are very subtle and easy to miss.
- However, if you know that your man is ready to have sex with you anytime, then you may be willing to experiment with acting on these illusive sparks. I call these subtle erotic feelings "the tiny voice of voracious desire."

## So if you want to have:

- The freedom to have sex anytime, without having to plan the tablet beforehand;
- A life free of the feeling that a pill is connected to sex;
- The freedom from judging yourself that you "need a pill" to have sex;

Then you would really enjoy the practice of taking DC; and this enjoyment can be experienced by both partners.

# Quickies

Why would anyone want quick sex?

How do you make a quickie satisfying?

When do you want to initiate a quickie?

## Quickies can be a great way to enjoy sex:

- When you feel a surge—or a whisper—of erotic turn on at the "wrong" time or place.
- When you want to create some excitement and fun *right now*.
- When you feel like you do not have the time for extended sex.
- When you feel that you don't have enough energy for sex.
- When—tell the truth—you are not that much into sex but want to be generous with your partner.
- When you want to generate some loving energy for yourself.

Quickies are sometimes judged as shallow or not meaningful or not the real thing. And certainly, it is good for couples to make time and spend time to connect on all the different levels. But let's not judge harshly, and let's be pragmatic about the benefits of quickies.

## Benefits of quickies:

Be honest: When was the last time that you and your partner had an extended love making session? If it has been a while, when was the last time that you had a quickie? Many couples find that it is so much better to have a quickie than nothing.

I would like you to consider that the quickie is not bad. Brief sexual play can give you fun and connection and sexual pleasure —and that's good! Sometimes it turns into a longer play session —and that's good too!

When the man in the relationship is taking Daily Cialis and is functioning well sexually, then the stage is set for quickies as well as long sessions. And the quickies work well as spontaneous sex. Although they can also be planned.

## Create what you want:

If there are a lot of quickies in your relationship, it is important to check in with yourself and with your partner periodically to make sure that you really are getting everything that you need. So you can identify what you want in your sexuality and incorporate that into your quickies. All of this goes for both women and men.

## What works for you for erotic play time?

Some women and some men get turned on quickly, and that is just fine. They do not have to pretend that they are different.

Some people take longer, and that is okay too, of course. They can even have a head start by starting solo. There is nothing wrong with the combination of masturbation and couple sex.

## Quickies and variety

They definitely do not need to be the same routine each time. It's a great time to try a new position, a new toy, or new way to play. You are doing it only for a short time so it's okay if you feel silly or if your back starts to ache.

## The big keys to making quickies successful:

- Be enthusiastic, or at least cooperative, with your partner's ideas.
- If their idea is not your favorite, you can always start planning how to do your favorite thing next time.
- Never ever make fun of your partner! Never be negative about what they say or want.
- Be generous with your partner. You are giving the gift of love to your partner which will be reflected back to you.
- Use the Daily Cialis regimen to give yourself and your partner the gift of spontaneity.
- You are building the relationship that you will live in. Take responsibility and take action to make it good.

# How to Do It: Taking Action

## Still Hesitant?

If the decrease of your erections is troubling you, and since Cialis and Daily Cialis are so safe and effective,

why would you not try it?

### Do you fear that once you take Cialis:

- You will get addicted to it?
  - o Actually, you will *not* get addicted to Cialis. This pill does not work like that. You can always decrease the dose or stop, with no problems.

- You will not able to function at all without it?

  - o Actually, your underlying function will *not* change.

- You will need ever increasing amounts of it to get the same effect?
  - o Actually, you will *not* need to take more to get the same effect.

- You should wait to take it as long as possible so you "don't use up your life time's supply to soon?"
  - o Actually, your body does *not* habituate to Cialis. It will continue to work for you. You do not "use it up."

- You will be walking around with a constant embarrassing erection?
    o Actually, you will *not* have out of control erections. You still need sexual stimulation to get hard. So you will still have control over when you are erect and when not.
- After taking it, you will feel: "I will never be the same again."
    o Actually, C does *not* change how you are as a person. You will still be exactly the same person that you always were.

## Which of these myths is holding you back?

- The myth that sex is shallow, so you shouldn't focus too much on it.
    o Actually, sex is important for physical and emotional well-being for you, your partner, and your relationship.
- The myth that you shouldn't "bother" your partner with sex at your age.
    o Actually, many older women love sex and miss it when it fades away, especially once they also find out how to make it work for them as they get older.
- The myth that suffering makes you a better human being.
    o Actually, you have suffered enough already. It is time for you to take action to be happy.
- The myth that it is good for you to finally have a lower sex drive and "more peace."

- o Actually, you know perfectly well that your sex drive is also a great source of life energy for you. Why would you want to live without that vital force?
- The myth that finally you have more heart connection, and less drive from your penis.
  - o Actually, guess what: You can have it all! You can have both the fire in the belly and the deep love in your heart. That is why I call it Best Sex Ever!

## Don't cave in to these sneaky deceptions:

- Puritanism is still alive and well in our society, unfortunately. Oddly, we may feel fear of fun, joy, and happiness.
- Our society disdains sex in older men. We call them "dirty old men."
- Is it more familiar for you to feel anxious and to suffer? Is it too uncomfortable or too scary to break out of that?

## Instead give yourself freedom:

- Look at yourself and notice how some of these subtle beliefs are present.
- You do not need to fight them—it is effective just to know that they are present.
- Look around you at the people and the society and notice these factors.
- You may choose to speak up out loud, or not.
- However, do speak up inside yourself against these thieves of your freedom.

- Remember that good rule: Question authority. Including your own.

## Do you have these needless worries?

- The fear of "putting something into my body"
- The fear that "Taking a pill is not natural."
- The fear of taking prescription medication
- The fear of taking something stronger than supplements
- The fear of needing to "detox" if I take this pill
- The fear that "It probably won't work, so why even try?"

## Actually:

- Cialis is effective for up to 85% of men, according to research studies.
- You won't know whether something works *for you* unless you try it.
- We are constantly putting substances into our bodies.
- Foods and supplements are substances too that affect our bodies.
- Whether a substance is a supplement or a prescription does not make it safer or riskier.
- You will *not* need to detox when taking this pill because your body already has effective ways for that.

## The clincher is: Cialis is good for you in many ways:

Not only is Cialis not bad for you,

- It is actually good for you in many different ways.
- It is beneficial for you in many *nonsexual* ways.

- It helps women and men function well at high altitude, like for hiking and skiing.
- It fights depression by three different mechanisms of action.
- It improves bladder and prostate symptoms in men.

For more information, check out the chapters on these topics.

## Look back over the contents of this book for:

- The chapters about too-low and too-high dosages.
- The chapters about safety and side effects and risks.
- The chapter on supplements.
- The chapters on sexual problems that apply to you.

For any other questions or concerns: Look at the list of chapter topics in the front of the book.

## It is my mission for you:

- To give you lots of information so you can make an informed decision.
- To be sure that you are safe.
- It could be that you have a feeling that Daily Cialis or Cialis or Viagra really are not for you.
- To help you question where that feeling is coming from and what it is based on.
- To help you and your doctor find the right dose for maximum good effects with minimum side effects.
- To prevent this: If you jump in *without* all the information from this book, you could use the wrong

dosage and get discouraged either by the side effects or by the lack of effectiveness.

## Always remember:

## You deserve You Best Sex Ever!

## You definitely can have Your Best Sex Ever!

- You will need to take action to reap the rewards.
- You will need to educate yourself to take charge of your sex life.
- You may need to step out of your comfort zone to try something new.
- Your future "you" will thank your present "you" for having created a better life for yourself.
- The reward of a rich life goes to those who are willing to take charge and try new things!

# Working With Your Doctor

Why is it important to find the right doctor for you?

What is the best way to approach your doctor?

How do you prepare for your doctor's visit?

## Find the right doctor for yourself and your problems!

- Find a doctor who is really experienced with these problems.
- Find someone who takes your situation seriously.
- Be willing to make the effort to find this doctor.
- Be willing to travel or have the visits via video conferencing.
- Be willing to spend the money.
- Learn the doctor's way of running their practice for optimal cooperation and convenience.
- Do not settle for someone who sells you a ton of supplements and a radical diet.
- Do not settle for someone who blames you for lack of progress.

## Imagine this unfortunate scenario:

- The middle-aged man finally goes to the doctor after procrastinating for months or even years.
- After hemming and hawing and talking about lots of other things, the patient says "By the way, doc, I have this problem with sex ..."

- And then the patient minimizes his sexual problem because it is so uncomfortable to talk about.
- Often the doctor is also uncomfortable talking about it.
- So the doctor may just use that phrase that I don't like, "At your age, that's how things are."
- Or the doctor may give the patients a prescription for Viagra or Cialis, with no information on how to take it optimally.
- Or the patient does not realize until later that something about the prescriptions is not optimal for him. But by then he is back in the cycle of procrastinating about going back to the doctor.

How much of this situation rings true to you?

## How to improve this scenario—
## The care and feeding of your doctor

Make the effort to create an effective relationship. Your doctor really does want to help you. It's just that they have so many different demands on them all the time. So you need to make it easy for them.

Usually it's best to have a private doc who knows you (or who kind of knows you, anyway). This medical doctor could be your urologist if you have one. Or they could be your internist or family doctor. It could also be a nurse practitioner or a physician's assistant.

Make an appointment. This appointment can be a yearly physical or a visit specifically for this purpose. When you are making the appointment, you will be asked about the purpose of your visit. If it is a yearly physical, that is easy. If you are coming in to request a Cialis prescription, then you might want to say something like "It is a private matter." Or you can just say that you want to talk about an issue with ED (erectile dysfunction).

Now that Viagra has been around so long and is so popular, more doctors are familiar with a conversation about ED. It is now a topic that is more routine for many doctors. So ED might be the easiest way to phrase your purpose for the visit.

You may have other interests for the Daily Cialis besides ED. However, you might consider sticking with the most familiar topic. Remember, we want to make this easy for the doctor. The doctors have keep up with so many topics that you can't expect them to know the fine points of DC. They might not even have heard of DC.

Medical people are usually curious and want to learn. Probably it would be useful to bring this book with you. For this purpose, a real paper copy works best. You might even give it to the doctor as a present. That way there is a good possibility that they will browse the book.

If they look at the book, it will help you in the future. And it will help other men. That is quite a good return on investment on the bucks you'll spend on the book. Doctors get few real gifts, so you will also make a favorable impression.

During the visit, get right to the point. Do not address other, more minor, concerns first because you are embarrassed. Talk about the most important topic first. Tell them what you want and why you want it. State the problem. Do not be subtle or understated. Do not minimize the problem. And state exactly what you would like them to do.

It is okay to have a clear idea of what strength tablets you want, how many you want to pick up from the pharmacy each time, and how many refills you want. It is okay to make that clear to the practitioner. Then you can ask whether they will write that prescription. Do your math ahead of time about the number and strength of pills so that you can give that information clearly.

You can talk to a pharmacist ahead of time to gather information about the cost to you, with your particular insurance plan. That way you can find out what will work for you financially. It would be a waste of your time to ask the doctor for a prescription that does not work for you financially.

By the time you read this, the brand name Cialis may have become available as generic tadalafil at a lower cost.

If the doctor is hesitant to write this prescription, ask—in a friendly voice—about the reasons for that. Do not use the word "Why?" It tends to make people defensive and makes them give answers that are less useful.

Instead, ask about concerns or needed information. They may have a medical concern about you and Cialis. You really do want to be safe, so you will want to listen to their concerns. They also may not be familiar with the concept of DC, and so they want to be cautious.

Stay positive and goal-oriented. Doctors really want to help patients who are nice to them and to their staff.

Typically, men do not want to complain or seem too dramatic. However, in a medical setting, being clear and strong about your problem gets more action. If you usually have a quiet and reserved style, you may get better results if you give dramatic illustrations of this problem's bad effects on your life.

# Make a Point of Being a Good Patient

- Come in often enough so the doctor feels like they know you.
- Don't come in too often if the doctor does not consider that necessary. You can just ask them about that.
- Have clear objectives for your visit.
- State your goals for the visit up front.
- Doctors get frazzled when they get "By the way, doc…" on their way out the door.
- Talk about your most important goal first.
- Do not bring in a lot of minor questions and problems that you could have looked up yourself.
- This doctor is not your therapist. If you bring up a lot of anxious emotions, then you will lose focus during the visit.
- Use your skills for effective meetings: Make sure that you have stated the next action step for both of you.
- Say "Thank you!" but don't be too effusive.
- Be concise. The doctor will be so grateful if you help them stay on schedule. It is very stressful to fall behind.
- Be nice to the staff.
- Know the office policies and follow them.
- Pay your bill promptly. If one pays at the time of the visit, be prepared for that.
- Ask them how they like to have refills handled for maximum ease for them.
- Give the office plenty of time for refills. Do not repeatedly or unnecessarily ask for rush service.

- On your prescription bottle, pay special attention to two items: How many refills are left. And also when those refills expire.

Doctors really do care about their patients. Make it easy for them to care for you. Ask for what you want, and be prepared to give information to back up your requests. Then you will be more likely to get what you want, and get it graciously.

# Dr. Erika's Medical Practice

What is it like to work with me as your doctor?

By now, you might be curious about what it is like to be a patient of mine.

## Here is how my medical practice works:

- My practice serves men locally in my Santa Barbara, CA, and Oakland,CA, offices.
- My practice also serves men anywhere in the USA with phone or videoconference appointments.
- My mission is: Getting midlife men back on top of their game, and keeping them there!
- More information at DrErikaMD.com.

## My expertise:

- Male midlife sexuality—problems and solutions
- Safe and effective use of DC, finely tuned for maximum impact
- Safe and effective use of testosterone, when indicated
- Optimizing male midlife sexual function
- Dealing with prostate problems
- Promoting glowing overall health
- Creating the synergy of testosterone and DC
- Use of DC for anti-aging benefits
- Use of DC for the nonsexual health benefits

## My attitude—I am:

- Non-judgmental.
- Extremely results-oriented.
- Easy to talk to about anything.
- "On your team."
- Committed to taking male sexual problems seriously.
- A doctor who gives lots of practical and user-friendly information.
- Informed on the topics that you want.

## I focus on optimal general health:

- Alleviating depressive and anxious moods
- Improving sleep
- Increasing energy
- Preserving muscle mass
- Promoting bone density

## Facets of my medical practice

All my patients are welcome to talk about anything they are curious about. Patients bring up a huge variety of topics. If a topic is outside my expertise, I usually have suggestions for resources.

Optimal sexual health includes enhancing the male libido as well as the quality of the erections and orgasms. To help the men to have their Best Sex Ever, we also talk about any sexual issues that they may have.

Working with me is one of the most important things that you can do for yourself, and also for the sake of your wife or girlfriend. This work has been proven to make relationships better. And research has shown that a relationship is a most important factor in your overall happiness. For men, it also is a major contributor to longevity with good quality of life.

This work with patients is not psychotherapy nor sex therapy. It is medical work with some coaching aspects.

We also focus on prostate health: Preventing and treating urinary prostate symptoms. This topic can be uncomfortable— even taboo—and yet it absolutely needs to be addressed. Here we talk about it in a relaxed and matter-of-fact way.

We want to prevent and improve bladder problems related to the prostate: Getting up at night to go to the bathroom, frequency, urgency, dribbling, sense of incomplete emptying, and needing to go again soon. These topics may not be easy or enjoyable to talk about, however they have major impact on your quality of life. If these problems affect your life right now, then they will be much worse ten to twenty years from now. In this case, investing in your future is very worthwhile. Your future self will seriously thank you for being proactive now!

Your prescription for Daily Cialis—if indicated for you—will not only turn the clock back on your sexual function and on your prostate symptoms but also give you improved moods, better relationships, and better all-around health.

Your prescription for testosterone—if indicated for you—gives you improved libido and the consequent happier outlook on life.

It can improve sexual function over the long run. It also increases your energy for working out and gives you better results from your work outs at the gym. It makes you more goal oriented and more confident. It even helps with prostate problems.

Remember that it can be useful to do a trial of DC or testosterone or both if they are indicated for you medically. You can take them for a few weeks or a few months and see for yourself how they work for you. Then you have really good information for making an informed decision.

You can always stop C or testo. You are never addicted. There are no negative consequences for starting DC or testo and then stopping it. So you can always do the experiment for yourself. So often in my office men say to me, "Thank you for giving me my life back!" That might be you saying that soon, if you take action.

## These are my goals for you:

- To feel sexy, young, vibrant, confident and masculine.
- To feel on top of your game in sex and in life.
- To feel sexually juicy and sexually confident.
- To have the satisfaction of your wife or girlfriend enjoying sex again.

## What my patients say:

- "You turned the clock back 20 years!"
- "It feels good to feel good."
- "Thank you for giving me my life back!"

- "I had forgotten how good it feels to feel good!"
- "You work not from an illness point of view but an improving-life point of view."
- "Thank you for the Best Sex Ever!"
- "I never expected to be having the Best Sex Ever at my age!"

It is my strong hope that you will invest in your well-being for now as well as for the future in these proven and effective ways.

# Dr. Erika: My Own Journey

My journey toward my current medical practice started in kindergarten.

My parents were psychotherapists. They were passionate psychologists. They lived and breathed their work all their lives. Both of them were constantly talking with each other and with me about various theories and practices of psychology since I was a child.

When I was in kindergarten, at dinner we would talk about Carl Jung because they both were in Jungian analysis. While I was in my teens they became fascinated by the human potential movement in California with Carl Rogers, with Alexander Lowen's Bioenergetics, with Esalen, with that heady mix of joy in the body and in spirit that all of these offered.

Then, during my time as a pre-medical student, I had the best study habits because my father had just added behavior modification to his repertoire.

During college, medical school, and my career, my personal extracurricular studies and learning were largely about various aspects of human psychology. My learning also incorporated systems therapy for couples and families, such as the family therapy of Virginia Satir.

My education has also included human sexuality in all its physiological, psychological, and philosophical aspects: the varieties of sexual expression, the problems, the solutions, the different ways of enhancing the sexual experience, as well as the spiritual and heart-centered aspects of sexuality, such as tantra.

So, while I am not a therapist or a sex therapist, my practice strongly includes psychological and sexological aspects.

When I am talking to my male patients, there is always awareness of their all-around well-being as well as their sexual vitality. And there is also an awareness of this man as part of a couple, and how best to support the happiness and the growth of the couple. You will notice this emphasis in this book.

Studies have shown that most of our happiness comes from our connections with the people around us, especially from our primary relationship. How things are going with our partner, wife, or girlfriend makes the biggest difference in how happy we are in life. So it is very much worth your while to continually make it your focus to cherish your partner, and to keep finding more ways to nourish her and the relationship.

So, after incorporating psychotherapy and sexology influences into my work, then came the hormones; to help my midlife patients more effectively I added bioidentical hormones to my practice, and my patients have benefited for many years now. All of these modalities help them feel really good in body, mind, emotion, and sexuality.

When my middle-aged patients come to me with problems, my attitude is that there is nothing wrong with them. The problem is just that due to the aging process, some of the necessary hormones for well-being have decreased. It is pure biology and physiology.

First my hormone practice was mostly for menopausal women. Then men also started to come to my office. A while back it became clear to me how middle-aged men are underserved for their midlife concerns. It has been, and continues to be, a fascinating process for me to learn about these complex creatures called men. I am constantly reading new research to study more and to apply it to their care.

Now my medical practice is specialized for midlife men only: To get them back on top of their game and to keep them there, to use the fascinating and effective concept of Daily Cialis for them. My goal is to optimize their mental, emotional, physical, and sexual functioning so that they continue to be in their prime for the years to come, and to accomplish that in safe, scientific, and effective ways.

Testosterone is a time-honored method. And now there is the concept of Daily Cialis, which is constantly evolving. DC has long lists of benefits both for optimal sexuality and for thriving all-around health.

This "Daily Cialis" book contains some of that information so that *you* can find ways to get back on top of your game. If you want to take it further and want information about my medical practice, please go to DrErikaMD.com.

It continues to be a frequent and gratifying experience for a man to say to me, "Dr. Erika, you have given me my life back!"

You can have that, too!

# How You Can Help Others

It continues to break my heart that so many midlife men suffer in silence. They really suffer a lot! And they suffer needlessly.

Almost every middle-aged man has issues ranging from ED and urinary problems to depressed moods and lack of confidence.

It is so sad to see the unhappiness because it is so easy, safe, and effective to improve these problems. And the methods work for almost everyone.

However, the men do not seem to realize that there are options. They do not appear to know that these problems can be fixed.

They do not seem to know that there are no bad consequences to the treatment: There is no price to pay for feeling On Top of Their Game.

The main reason for this lack of information is that men do not talk to each other about these topics. Each man thinks that he is the only one, and that there is something wrong with him, and he should "man up" and not complain.

When I had women patients (now I specialize only in men), the women would talk to each other. They would refer their friends and relations to me. Women do share this kind of information.

You are lucky that you ran across this book. Then you took action for your better future by buying this book. Help the men around you to be lucky too. It's easy: It is completely socially acceptable to recommend a book.

So for the men who are your friends, relations, co-workers, fellow gym rats: Give them the gift that will change their lives. Tell them about this book. Recommend this book. Show them this book. Lend them this book. Buy a few copies as gifts.

To keep that conversation light, you just say something like "Great stuff in this book. Turns back the clock. Really works."

Tell your doctors about the book. Better yet: Do your good deed for the day and give them a copy to benefit you and the other men in their practice.

Women also need this information. Sometimes it is easier to talk to a woman, to give her the book recommendation. Women care about their husband or boyfriend's health, so they will want to read it. Often the best way to help men is to educate the women.

Show the men and women around you how much you care: Turn them on to this information! Your generosity will give them their life back.

What would it take for you to give them that leg up?

So they too can have Best Sex Ever—just like you will too!

# The Cost of This Medical Care

The good life—and the good sex life—do carry a cost. Yes, it does cost something to buy the Cialis. And it costs more to add the testosterone. Then there are the charges for the knowledgeable and experienced doctor who takes care of you.

Nevertheless, once men realize how much better their life has become, then the costs are not a problem for them. They are happy to pay to get the things that money cannot buy: their juicy sexuality, a better marriage, and feeling younger, happier, and more confident. How much is it worth to you to be in your prime for yourself and your partner?

Usually this kind of medical care by this type of doctor is not covered by insurance. Doctors like me often have just a small practice. We focus on the patient care, not on running a big office with lots of staff. That also means that we do not have the staff to process insurance paperwork. The men typically pay cash out of pocket for this kind of doctor.

However, be sure to spend your money only on the things that you give you the most bang for your buck: Doctor's visits and Cialis. Maybe testosterone. Then it could actually be less of an expense than buying lots of different supplements and treatments.

Be careful: You can spend a lot of money on all kinds of supplements and powders and diets and treatments that promise dramatic sexual effects. You'd likely be wasting your time and your money. Better to go for the tried and true.

Also be careful: Choose your doctor wisely so that you get expert advice about the safety, efficacy and optimal dosing of Cialis and testosterone for you.

## Good news about generic pricing:

By the time you read this, in addition to brand name Cialis, the generic tadalafil may be on the market, or it will be soon. The generic is expected to be significantly lower in cost.

At the time of this writing, in addition to brand name Viagra, generic sildenafil is starting to be available. Keep checking on websites that compare drug prices such as GoodRx.

Be aware that it is possible that some strengths of sildenafil - such as 20mg - may be available as inexpensive generic. However some of the other strengths - such as 25mg or 50mg or 100mg - may still be full price. When you compare prices, be really clear of the strengths in mg that you are checking, so that you are not comparing apples and oranges.

Also be careful about which medication you are checking since both sildenafil and tadalafil now come in 20mg tablets.

## Think about the big picture:

- Where can you spend your money that will have greater immediate as well as long-lasting effects on the quality of your life?
- What else brings you more joy in life than enjoying your Best Sex Ever?

# Dr. Erika's Courses

To keep your Best Sex Ever coming:

Please check my website for courses, books, and other offerings.

DrErikaMD.com

## Dr. Erika's Online Courses:
## Fun, sexy, and chock-full of info:

- Best Sex Ever! Men's Midlife Health and Sexuality
- The Best Sex Ever nonDiet: How to eat lightly for effective weight management while enjoying life and sex. Shape your body for love! Love your body!
- The Best Sex Ever! Happiness Infrastructure Project
- The Best Sex Ever! Singles and Relationship Course

## Future topics:

- How to plan and create a sexual date night that works
- How to be a male sexual super star
- How to have the Best Sex Ever in midlife
- How to have spontaneous sex in midlife
- Things that the midlife woman can do to have the Best Sex Ever for herself
- What does it take—for a man—to be ready for sex anytime?
- What does it take—for a woman—to be ready for sex anytime?
- Supplements and hormones for sex

- The Female Low Desire course

**Please email me: Which topics interest _you_?**

Made in USA - North Chelmsford, MA
1043827_9781671279995
01.14.2020 1507